Beyond *the* Edge

Beyond the Edge

One woman's journey out of
post-natal depression and anxiety

Hazel Rolston

ivp

INTER-VARSITY PRESS
Norton Street, Nottingham NG7 3HR, England
Email: ivp@ivpbooks.com
Website: www.ivpbooks.com

First published 2008
Reprinted 2008

British Library Cataloguing in Publication Data
A catalogue record for this book is available from the British Library.

ISBN 978-1-84474-216-5

Set in Chaparral 11.5/14pt
Typeset in Great Britain by CRB Associates, Reepham, Norfolk
Printed and bound in Great Britain by Ashford Colour Press, Gosport,
Hampshire

Inter-Varsity Press publishes Christian books that are true to the Bible and that
communicate the gospel, develop discipleship and strengthen the church for its
mission in the world.

Inter-Varsity Press is closely linked with the Universities and Colleges Christian
Fellowship, a student movement connecting Christian Unions in universities
and colleges throughout Great Britain, and a member movement of the
International Fellowship of Evangelical Students. Website: www.uccf.org.uk

To those who feel lost in rough terrain
and held captive by Despair

Contents

Acknowledgments

First of all, I would like to thank my agent, Pieter Kwant, Sue Prior and the staff at Piquant; Eleanor Trotter, my editor, and all who have been commissioned by IVP to assist in the publication of this book (in particular Helen Birkbeck, for her copy-editing skills and careful honing of the text); and all the other valued contacts who kindly read my manuscript. Without your vision, belief and feedback this book would not have been written, nor its hope made explicit.

Secondly, I would like to thank everyone who has encouraged me throughout the writing process: most of all, my family and friends, who listened graciously to the highs and lows of my literary regurgitation. I would also like to give a special 'thank you' to Jennifer Rees Larcombe who has inspired and encouraged me to write this book and who supported me in prayer throughout. My gratitude goes also to the staff at Café Kondi, who cheered me on over delicious cappuccinos; Wesley Owen employees in Bristol and Bath who encouraged me to continue on my way; and the people at Trinity Theological College (some of whom ministered to me unwittingly through their chapel worship as I worked in the library). In addition, I would like to thank those within my church and others who have prayed for me through this process.

I would also like to acknowledge all those who have supported me, in any way, throughout my life, even if it appears in this book that my needs were not fully met at the time: thank you for trying to help. Now, with a clearer perspective, I am able to appreciate that you *did* reach out to me and give me what you could at the time. I bring up uncomfortable topics now only because I believe them to be linked to untouched wider issues in the church; I do not mention them in order to apportion blame or score points. If I should even try to point the finger at any individual's failure towards me, there would be three fingers pointing back representing those I have equally failed!

Others I would particularly like to thank are my parents, for their commitment to nurturing my faith, and their relentless love and generous support over the past forty plus years, and also my wider family and friends for the different ways in which you have helped me. I mentioned few by name in this book, but that by no means belittles your contribution. Many of you who remain anonymous supported me through my darkest hours: thank you for that.

Finally, there are three who have been constantly with me through my most difficult days, and to them I give my deepest love and gratitude. First, my daughter, 'Katherine'. I have changed your name for your protection, but you know who you are! Your laughter, perseverance and character have inspired me to live amid life's challenges, and my love for you has driven me on to seek God and be the best mother I could be for you. Nurturing you and watching you grow is such a blessing to me. You are wonderful.

Steve – what can I say? You have been amazing, better than I could ever have hoped for or dreamed of. Thank you for supporting me in writing this book, and, more importantly, for sharing in the darkness of my wild place and not

abandoning me to my rough terrain. Thank you for supporting me in so many ways, not least through your belief that a
brighter road awaited us.

Finally, God. Thank you for your faithfulness and the
blessings you have given me, even though at times I could
not see them, for providing me with enough sustenance to
recognize and resist the voice of Despair, and for helping me
find my way out of his shadow. Thank you for showing
me that, through your grace, you love us, just as we are!

Foreword

I first met Hazel when she was nine years old. Her family had come over to England from Northern Ireland to attend a Christian house party we were helping to run. My husband and I were in charge of the children's activities, and Hazel stands out vividly in my memory while most of the rest of the children are forgotten. She was a beautiful child, with big blue eyes, long blonde hair and an engaging smile. During the day she seemed happy and carefree, but how she hated going to bed at night! She simply could not sleep. I used to babysit to allow all the parents to have their evenings free, and I would sit on Hazel's bed for hours while she told me what it was like to live in Northern Ireland at the height of 'the Troubles'.

'Bombs often go off in our town,' she told me, her eyes round with fear. 'I'm scared when my daddy goes to work that he'll never come back.'

Years later I met Hazel again at a retreat I was running in Bristol for young mothers. She had grown into a beautiful woman, and we laughed and reminisced over a meal. She was at the height of her anxiety and depression at the time, but later, when she told me this, it was hard to believe because she concealed her pain so well, behind that same beautiful smile. I guess an awful lot of us do exactly the same!

Since then we have kept in touch by post and then e-mail, and we've met at writers' courses and conferences. Hazel often told me how much she longed to write a book, but at the same time she shrank away from embarking on this one. When she finally dared to begin, we e-mailed often, so I know only too well how much it cost her to relive memories she would rather have forgotten.

Last week I read the final manuscript, and found it a deeply moving experience. Not only was it a gripping story about someone I know and respect, but I found it very helpful on a personal level. For the last nine months I have had to watch someone very close and dear to me going through an episode of acute anxiety and depression such as Hazel describes so vividly. The book helped me to understand the mental torture this kind of illness produces so that I was much better equipped to do the things that help, and avoid the things that definitely do not!

I believe this book will also help me in my job as a counsellor. I frequently see clients who are suffering from reactive or post-natal depression and also those suffering from acute stress. Few of them are as articulate as Hazel. They want to explain to me how they feel but the illness itself often makes that impossible. Because Hazel has dared to write this book so graphically, I feel much better equipped to help them. So many of them, like Hazel, also find that their Christian friends, and even church leaders, are unable to offer support to people going through mental illness.

It is only fair to warn you that this book is not a comfortable read. In fact, whether you are a sufferer or a carer, you may find it deeply painful at times. Yet I strongly believe that the Christian world needs to understand the horrors of an illness like this and be better equipped to help. So I can recommend this book highly, not only to sufferers but also to their families, friends and church leaders as well as their counsellors and professional carers. I believe that when you have finished reading it you will want to join me in saying a most sincere 'thank you' to Hazel for her courage in writing this very special book.

Jennifer Rees Larcombe
November 2007

Introduction

Does God know our limits? Will he let us be tried beyond what we can bear, or will he provide a way out so we can endure our suffering? Even in my darkest moments, I never doubted that God was with me. Yet in some ways this made me feel worse! Why would he not rescue me when I knew he *could*?

When our ten-week-old daughter suffered a cardiac arrest, I instantly felt pushed *beyond the edge*, where I became lost and cut off by the fog of anxiety and severe post-natal depression.[1] There I experienced deep, passionate emotions, which forced me to face questions I would rather have ignored.[2] This book is about my struggle to leave that rough terrain behind while confronting deep spiritual issues.

Until my descent into depression, I had always been able to sort out my theological questions by listening to the teaching in my church services and through housegroup Bible study and personal reading. Struck down by a post-viral illness many years ago, I was able to rely on God by 'journaling' my prayers and by sensing the presence of God in the absence of immediate theological answers. However, when I encountered acute anxiety and post-natal depression, all these things became inaccessible to me.

So how do you maintain your faith when you are suffering from an illness that removes all clarity of thought and demolishes any chance of *feeling* the hope of your faith, or sensing God? *You hang on to what you know to be true, even though you do not see or feel it personally!* This was what kept me trusting God and practising my faith throughout my anxiety and post-natal depression: my knowledge and experience of God before my illness. Thus, when the grim voice of Despair offered me the path of suicide, I knew God had not planned that route for me. Even though I could not see it, there had to be another way out. However, I needed sustenance to maintain that stance, something I found through medical help, family, friends and prayer, to mention but a few.

Through this book I long to pass on to you what I have discovered: not a formula for instant escape or a prayer guaranteed to get you out of your messy place, but rather my belief that 'God *is* faithful and he will not let you be tempted beyond that you can bear, but when you are tempted he will also provide a way out so that you can endure it'.[3] The way out may seem totally obscured by the fog of your anxiety or depression, but nevertheless I believe it is there.

However, even after we have left our depression, the way forward may seem unrecognizable, overshadowed by darkness. Injuries from my wild place meant that I was unable to climb to all the lofty heights of my desires and so, initially, I struggled to walk along the path that was accessible to me. Again, I was visited by Despair, who tried to entice me onto his path of destruction. However, as I now look back from a different place, I am so glad that I did not follow him but kept travelling in pursuit of God.

It is my hope that through sharing my story you too will see that, no matter how bad you feel or how wild and messy your life is, *all is not lost*: God can bring new life out of rough places. Often I have asked him, 'Why have you given *me* the

opportunity to write my story? I am not a model Christian.'
To which he has replied, 'Because your story shows that
I remain faithful, even to my prickly, wounded people
"beyond the edge".'

Hazel Rolston
November 2007

1 Over the edge

Like an open book, you watched me grow from conception
    to birth;
All the stages of my life were spread out before you,
The days of my life all prepared
Before I'd even lived one day.
(Psalm 139:16, *The Message*)

Katherine was blue. She wasn't breathing and, as I looked at her, my head felt as if it had received a massive blow. Our ten-week-old baby was lying motionless and I could hardly believe my eyes. A nurse ushered us out of the room and I looked upwards and spoke silently: 'God, I thought you knew me! You have allowed me to be pushed beyond what I can bear.'

My husband, Steve, and I stood howling in the corridor as the crash bell rang out. Medics ran from all directions and it felt as if we were part of a melodramatic TV show. Our only child was fighting for her life and we did not care whom we upset by our very obvious grief. Steve collapsed and had to be helped into a side room. I knelt beside him, and although semi-upright felt as though I too was horizontal, that this recent blow had pushed me right over the edge. It was unbelievable to think that, after all we had come through, we were going to lose Katherine.

* * *

Katherine had arrived in this world on a Tuesday in May 1997, following a thirty-six-hour labour. I had felt so relieved when her delivery ended smoothly. Being an ex-nurse with some midwifery experience, I had feared a last-minute hitch, as I had learnt not to take anything for granted. I had harboured secret fears that I would not have the 'right' maternal feelings for my baby at birth, so was very relieved to discover that from the very outset I felt hugely protective towards her. I knew instinctively that her survival was now the most important thing in the world. Initially she progressed well, despite a little jaundice. She fed and slept regularly and we seemed to be adapting easily to family life.

However, two weeks after her birth the 'honeymoon' ended. Without warning, Katherine started to cry a lot. It did not seem like classic colic,[1] and as time went on she cried even more. Basic tasks were too much to manage: we regularly had to stop eating, or abort walks with her in the pram, as she writhed and screamed too much for us to continue. Night-times were particularly difficult, as she slept for only short periods at a time. Meanwhile, other new mums were telling me that things were getting easier: their babies were sleeping longer at night and developing predictable behaviour. Steve and I wondered why Katherine was not settling.

In the midst of all this, fresh allegations were made against me in an ongoing complaint procedure at work. As a social worker, I had faced an incredibly difficult dilemma. Consequently, when the health visitor arrived, I was feeling like an emotional and physical wreck. I explained that I was feeling overwhelmed with worry, but she seemed too nice to understand and appeared shocked and even scared by my honesty. She gave me a questionnaire which asked me if I doubted my ability to mother, if I was more tearful than usual, and if I was feeling isolated. After answering 'yes' to most questions, I was declared depressed and told to visit my doctor.

I duly went to see my GP, who said she was not sure whether I was depressed or just totally worn out by the various pressures I was under. She gave me a prescription for antidepressants but recommended that I wait a few days, to see how things went, before starting them. The next day I was feeling a little better, so I decided not to bother. But Katherine continued to be very unsettled and I became convinced that there was something terribly wrong with her. The same message kept coming back to me: 'She has colic.' Then, one day at the weighing clinic, another health visitor said curtly, 'Maybe you need to look at why you cannot cope with a crying child', and I began to believe that the problem was mine.

Despite my doubts, I rang the on-call doctor one evening when Katherine was seven weeks old, as she had been shrieking for a long time after I had changed her nappy. Steve and I raced round the corner to the doctor's surgery, arriving with Katherine looking settled by the car journey. The doctor examined her, but then, smiling sweetly, pointed out to us that it was very normal for a baby to cry a lot in the first three months of its life, though for us, as first-time parents, it probably seemed very unusual. I left feeling angry and frustrated that our concerns had not been taken seriously.

Then, all of a sudden, Katherine's crying stopped completely. 'She has just settled down, like my friends' babies,' I told myself, 'but why the dramatic change?' I wondered, not realizing that the drama had yet to start!

Steve, Katherine and I enjoyed a couple of peaceful days and nights before the vomiting began. It started one Saturday evening. We were watching TV and eating a takeaway when we heard Katherine making strange noises through the baby-listening device. I raced upstairs to find her vomiting profusely, lying in copious amounts of undigested milk which had instantly spread from the cot to the floor. I yelled at Steve to come quickly. She continued to be very sick. At 4 am, when she vomited up some green bile, I rang the on-call GP. He said it was probably just a tummy bug and that I should take her to her own doctor on Monday. I brought her into our bed but she continued to vomit everything I breastfed her.

By 10 am, Steve and I were very worried. We felt torn between obeying the doctor's advice and ringing him again. Sitting in the living room with Katherine on my knee, I noticed her breathing had changed: it was laboured and unlike earlier. She was becoming drowsy and difficult to feed. Despite not wanting to make a fuss, I rang the out-of-hours GP surgery again and a duty doctor asked me to bring her straight there.

Steve and I scrambled round the house and dressed in the previous day's clothes, not taking time to shower. In the car I scolded myself for not having bathed Katherine before leaving. Her cradle cap was unsightly and I feared being labelled a neglectful, depressed mother.

Despite the fact that Katherine was sick all down my orange and lime shirt, I was worried that I was making a fuss over a tummy bug and that I was going to be told off for wasting the doctor's time. I had lost confidence in my skills as a parent, as professionals kept dismissing me. I wondered if I could trust the instinct that told me that something was seriously wrong.

The GP listened carefully and, much to our surprise, validated our concerns. She said that she thought this was something more serious than a stomach virus and that we should take Katherine straight to the children's Accident and Emergency Department. It was a Sunday morning and, as we drove to the hospital, I thought of all my friends in church, listening to the sermon before going through to drink coffee and socialize. They were having such a different morning, blissfully unaware that our lives were unravelling before our very eyes. God and everyone we knew so well seemed a million miles away and how I yearned for my family and friends in my native Ireland, as I still felt we were so unknown and insignificant in Bristol.

The staff at the Children's Hospital seemed quite relaxed about Katherine, but I became defensive when they asked me whether I had taken time to give her colic preparations and wind her properly. We had both spent so many hours pacing the floor and giving her all the colic preparations on the market that I was furious at the slightest insinuation of neglect.

After a while Katherine was taken for an X-ray, and the doctor reported that they could see only part of her bowel in the picture and she needed a scan. He still seemed relaxed and said that maybe the lack of a clear image meant she had a lot of air in her bowel. Halfway through the scan, I realized there was a bigger problem when the radiologist started asking me questions that set alarm bells screaming in my ears: 'Did you have any scans when you were pregnant? When did you have your last scan?'

I started to panic, as I could sense bewilderment on the part of the medical staff and dreaded what they were going to tell us. We were taken upstairs to a waiting area, the curtain was drawn round and the doctor pulled up a chair. 'We have discovered that your daughter was born with a diaphragmatic hernia, which has now obstructed,' he said. Despite being a qualified nurse, I had no idea what he was talking about, and just could not take it in due to sheer terror. 'This means she was born with a hole in her diaphragm and now almost all of her bowel has protruded through the hole. The bowel has probably been going in and out of the hole over the past weeks and, now that it is stuck, the pain has eased but she cannot digest or process feeds. The bowel has stopped working and this is causing vomiting. She needs immediate surgery to rectify this.'

All I could hear was 'needs immediate surgery'. I was dumbstruck. While feeling some relief that there was after all an explanation for the mayhem of the previous weeks, I also felt horrified at the thought of Katherine enduring a major operation. Unable to gauge the seriousness of the problem, I asked if she would return to Intensive Care. The doctor's evasiveness told me that this would indeed be a serious and risky operation.

Things progressed quickly and within an hour we were asked to carry Katherine into the anaesthetic room. Kissing her goodbye was heartbreaking. I left crying, with Steve consoling me. While waiting, we took the opportunity to ring our family and friends. I longed for someone we knew to be there, to put their arms around us and share in our fear and pain. I felt very alone. Life outside the hospital walls seemed remote and irrelevant.

It was an immense relief when, a few hours later, Katherine returned to the ward, awake and comfortable, albeit attached to loads of drips and monitors. We heard from the consultant that the operation had gone very well, and that her diaphragm had been intact except for one hole, which they had now stitched up. The consultant seemed so upbeat and optimistic that I felt sure that the worst was over. Steve and I went to sleep in our hospital bed, believing that a difficult chapter had ended and thanking God for saving our daughter.

The next morning I woke at 4 am and needed to express some breast milk. I decided to do it on the ward, where I could also check on Katherine's progress. I suggested to Steve that he should sleep on, as I thought we might need to stagger our visits later in the day, and take turns to sleep.

When I arrived, Katherine was crying and a nurse was trying to make her comfortable. My heart ached for her as she lay there, so small, separated from us and surrounded by machines. The nurse suggested that I hold her. She took off all Katherine's monitors, as she said that she was progressing really well and no longer needed them. I was delighted and started to feel confident that we had turned a positive corner.

I was nursing Katherine when Steve arrived at half past seven. The doctors were due to start their rounds and we decided not to stay as we had already talked to them at length the night before. Instead, we planned to walk the mile to our home, shower, have breakfast and return in a couple of hours. We were starving, as we had hardly eaten anything in the past twenty-four hours, and I in particular smelt rather sicky!

Just as we were getting up to leave, the anaesthetist arrived and asked about Katherine's recovery. I told him that she seemed to be doing well, although she appeared to be in some pain. His reply that this was to be expected seemed defensive, but then he said he would give her some extra epidural[2] to relieve it. He pushed some extra fluid up the syringe that was attached to her epidural needle and instructed the nurse to give her paracetamol and take five-minute observations. Now, as an ex-nurse, I knew that five-minute observations were taken only when there was a fairly high level of risk. Instinctively we stayed with Katherine and postponed any notion of breakfast or a shower.

Steve and I stood by her cot and within a minute noticed that her dummy had fallen out of her mouth. I immediately thought this was strange and went to fetch the nurse. Walking quickly, I tried to remember the risks of epidurals and wondered whether it had just slowed down her breathing. I hoped I was not going to make a fuss or interrupt anyone. When the nurse and I returned to the ward, we found Steve dumbfounded and Katherine blue. She had stopped breathing and her heart had stopped beating. The stages of my daughter's life were spread open before God[3] and I feared I had seen all of them.

The bombshell I had been waiting for all my life had finally arrived.

2 Learning to ride on a bumpy road

I tell you the truth, anyone who will not receive the kingdom of God like a little child will never enter it.

(Luke 18:17)

My life's journey began in May 1963, when I, a tiny redhead, entered a loving Protestant Northern Irish family. I was born in a cottage hospital in Lisburn, a thriving market town eight miles from Belfast. Northern Ireland was at peace, at least on the surface, as the undercurrents that led to 'the Troubles'[1] did not fully emerge until six years later.

I grew up in the countryside, three miles from Lisburn, with my parents and two older brothers. My paternal grandmother and two aunts lived behind our home, and uncle, aunt and cousins lived 'across the field'. It was a Christian community, where giving one's life to God was to be admired rather than scorned, and so believing in God became an integral part of my life.

My father co-owned a family department store with his brother and cousin, where they sold carpets, furniture, toys and many household goods. I spent my early years mostly under my mother's care, as she had given up her career in clothing design to nurture our family. Born in Northern Ireland, she had moved to Dublin as a child, where she was brought up as a Quaker. Later she returned north of the border and became a Presbyterian when she married my father.

Initially, I developed in a carefree world of outdoor sport and imaginary games, with my brothers and three male cousins as willing playmates. Much of my time was spent playing football and cricket and making dens in the garden. I was fortunate in that we had a lovely house to live in: comfortable, but not pretentious, as my parents' Christian values permeated our home, so that we had what we needed, rather than what we wanted. Despite seeing many luxury items in my father's shop, I grew up to respect my parents' attitude of restraint from indulging in available material pleasures, and so, with the exception of birthdays and Christmas, I learned to expect the same of myself.

I started nursery when I was three years old and enjoyed the company of my new friends. I was already developing a strong sense of justice and an awareness of others' needs. On one occasion, when a new girl arrived and others ganged up against her, I was appalled at their cruelty and insisted that she be included in our games. I attribute this early display of altruism to my parents' values. Being a Quaker, my mum had a strong sense of equality, of everyone being the same in God's eyes. Combined with my dad's generosity and community spirit, this developed in me a core thread of empathy and fairness.

From reception, I went to a private prep school, where I learnt to read and write in a small and intimate setting. There I discovered a love of creative writing and an innate satisfaction in creating my own literary order. I claimed from an early age that I was going to write books when I grew up. However, that desire was almost snuffed out before being revived in later years.

For as long as I could remember, our home had been used in Christian service. My parents hosted residential camps and 'squashes', where as many young people as possible (up to a hundred-plus) squeezed in to hear the gospel or talks on Christian discipleship from a visiting speaker. Although my parents never preached, they were effective and skilled hosts. There was an excitement in the air every month as the house was being prepared, and I loved sneaking out of bed and looking over the banisters at the young people who overflowed onto the stairs. Although familiar with the idea that the Christian message needed to be shared, it wasn't until I understood it for myself that I decided to commit my life to God.

We visited my mother's parents in Dublin every Easter, and on one occasion I asked my mother what the festivities were all about. She explained that Easter was a time when Christians celebrate the resurrection of Jesus, after his death on the cross over 2,000 years ago. She told me that God loved me so much that he had allowed his only Son, Jesus, to die for me, and that Jesus' death made it possible for me to find forgiveness for the things I had done wrong so I could go and live with God at the end of my life. I felt very moved by this revelation and immediately prayed a prayer of commitment to follow Christ. I envisaged God as a kind but distant figure, someone who was trying to create a world order through huge personal sacrifice, and I instinctively wanted to help. I took it all very seriously and allowed it to infiltrate my play, insisting on being the teacher and getting my unsuspecting friends to read Christian children's books as schoolwork!

So my life's journey started with ease. At the end of my infant education, aged seven, I won the all-round cup for best personal achievement at sports day and was an optimistic and happy child. It was as if I had been given all the tools I needed to develop well, all the physical resources

I needed – like the gift of a new bike, with family representing stabilizers, and faith representing my vision for the future. Initially the road was smooth, my environment was without challenge, and I enjoyed holding my head up high and freewheeling as a carefree young rider. Little did I know that the surface of the path was about to change and soon I would be struggling to balance my vehicle along an uneven road!

My perspective on life changed gradually rather than in obvious response to one event. I started to become aware of daily tragedies. I would hear on the radio at breakfast and during the teatime news that people were being killed and maimed daily by bombs within our small province. My regular journeys to and from school became chequered with the presence of armed police and army convoys. Often I felt bewildered as we queued in traffic and a soldier pointed his gun straight into our car from his jeep in front. 'Our town has become a very dangerous place to live,' I thought to myself.

Gradually I became wary of separation from my family in case we should be caught in an incident while apart from one another. One evening at a friend's house I could not get to sleep, so I got up and sat with the adults for a while. I became very, very anxious and started to experience a deep dread that something terrible was going to happen. The ten o'clock news came on TV and fuelled my fears, and two hours later I insisted that I be allowed to go home. It was many years before I felt able to leave my family at night again.

Lisburn itself, a large, mainly Protestant town, and home to a British Army base, was sometimes the target of sectarian bombings that injured civilians on both sides of the community. It was certainly not the worst area of Northern Ireland, but to my childish mind it felt like the front line. As 'the Troubles' progressed, killings of people on both sides of the community escalated, and shops in my hometown became a target for bombings. As a key-holder, my father was responsible for checking his premises in the event of a bomb scare in Lisburn. Often we would be sitting eating our evening meal and a subtitled message would be displayed on the TV screen: 'BOMB ALERT! WOULD ALL KEY-HOLDERS IN THE LISBURN AREA PLEASE RETURN TO THEIR PREMISES TO SEARCH FOR DEVICES'.

Consequently, I would feel unable to relax all evening. I hated my dad going out to search for bombs in his shop and I felt terrified that I would never see him again. I went up to my bedroom and looked out of my window at the lights of Lisburn and hoped that I would not hear a bomb or see smoke. Often I had to go to bed before Dad came back. The worst thing was when the phone rang in the middle of the night and I would hear Dad answering, 'OK, I will come now' and then hear him walking about. I would ask what was wrong. 'There's a bomb scare in Lisburn; I have to go and check the shop; I'm sure it's nothing,' Dad would say. Sitting hugging my blanket, I would watch him drive off into the night. I would sit and watch for as long as I could, hoping that he would return.

My fears for our safety increased when 'the Troubles' entered our own back yard – literally. It was an ordinary day and delivery lorries and cars were driving in and out of the back yard of my father's shop. While at school, I heard a large bomb go off, causing our community to shudder into silence before the inevitable emergency sirens. Word came through that a bomb had gone off in the town, half a mile away, but that nobody had been killed. We all sighed with relief. But later I discovered that the bomb had gone off in my dad's shop, and I was very scared and upset. One employee had been seriously injured and had lost an arm and a leg in the blast, as the bomb had detonated shortly after a car had been driven out of the yard. This war now began to feel personal. Our family business had been targeted because

Protestants owned it, and this meant someone knew my dad was a Protestant and meant to hurt him because of it.

I dreaded going to bed, as the quiet darkness made my fears reverberate around my mind. I did not know what was wrong with me, but I just could not get to sleep and feared yet another night of lying awake until the early hours. Each night I made Mum promise to visit me before she went to bed. Then we agreed a time when I could wake her if I was still unable to sleep. Sometimes I fell asleep and other times I did not, but paced the dimly-lit landing waiting for time to pass. When the appointed hour arrived, I was wracked with guilt. A sensitive child, I could see that my mum and dad had enough worries of their own and I did not want to bother them with my insomnia. Sometimes I was able to talk myself back into bed, but other times I carefully dodged the creaky floorboards across my parents' bedroom floor.

'What's wrong?' Mum would ask.

'I can't sleep,' I would say, and then she would get up and climb into my bed, so as not to wake my dad. I became dependent on reassurance from Mum, as if it was the chain on my bike and without it I would meet a collision. I could no longer look around, go off-road or try an unmarked route. I lacked confidence that I could manage my bike or reach a destination on my own. I could cope with only the safest, easiest route possible. I began to feel a failure as I watched others speed by. I stopped enjoying sport. I began to fail at school and refused to go on trips away with friends. My aim was to follow my family wherever they rode. I would look neither left nor right. My road felt very uneven, as if there were potholes round every corner. It required my full attention to keep my balance, riding along on my bumpy road.

My world became reduced. Its limits were all too evident to me when, aged eleven, I refused to take part in the sports day that I had previously won. I recognized that I felt completely different now, ruled by internal constrictions to 'live safely, not take risks and reduce the chance of something bad happening'. Less movement reduced my chance of injury.

In 1974 I found out that I had failed my eleven-plus, the entrance exam that allowed me free passage into the adjoining grammar school. My parents were supportive and told me not to worry. One of my brothers had previously failed his eleven-plus but within a year had passed his review, an assessment test which granted similar scholarship status to the eleven-plus. However, I feared that I would not follow in his footsteps and would cause my parents financial hardship. One year later my fears were realized. In the 1,000-pupil grammar school I slipped into the bottom ranks for all subjects and my belief in my own stupidity was born.

Simultaneously 'the Troubles' escalated, so education and my long-term future began to feel irrelevant. 'Sure, I could be blown up at any time,' I thought, and I gave up trying to build for my future. Instead, I took a hedonistic perspective and concentrated on enjoying life moment by moment. This was hard for my parents as it meant I stopped working at school. I milked my innocent looks and began cheating or messing around instead, as I was frightened of discovering how incapable I really was. In geography tests, instead of labelling the maps I would colour them in. In history, I would draw ancient pictures or doodle, and in maths I resorted to writing words rather than numbers!

One day, our maths teacher told us that our class were so stupid that we would be better off helping terrorists than sitting in his room – i.e. if *we* helped them, their plans would fail! He suggested that during our test we should write words like 'Demis Roussos' rather than numbers, as our numerical answers were always wrong! My friend and I thought we would do this for a laugh, so instead of trying to answer the test correctly we repeatedly wrote down the name of this famous singer. While the teacher was collecting the papers, he uncharacteristically said that if we did not 'do reasonably badly' he would send our papers to the headmaster. Panic! So much so that we turned round and asked for help from two girls who were sitting behind us. However, to make matters worse, we were caught cheating, and our tests were collected before we had the opportunity to remove 'Demis Roussos'. I returned home that evening in trepidation, but it was a few days before the test paper actually arrived (for which, incidentally, I achieved a minus mark). When I got home, Mum had written me a letter telling me how disappointed she was with my behaviour. That night I ate my tea politely with our American guest, fearing that when she left my life would end. But there were no great repercussions that evening, just an ache in my heart for getting caught and letting my parents down.

Unknown to us all, my rebellion concealed a frightened and angry child. I was frightened by life and angry that my parents could not make it better for me. My life felt futile and I wanted to escape the terror that surrounded me. School was the one place where I felt safe, as I reckoned that even the terrorist groups would not bomb a school, and I wanted to enjoy it rather than toil for a life I might never have.

The only way I could manage my insurmountable fears was to push them down and deny their presence. I felt like a rabbit that had been cornered. There was an inevitability about my fate: I would either die prematurely in 'the Troubles' or live as a failure, for my inability to achieve at school strengthened my belief in my stupidity. Even my faith failed to give me the answers I needed. Indeed, it seemed to add further restrictions to my already small world.

I decided I wanted to be a Bay City Roller! I wanted to dress up, have a laugh and enjoy myself, be outrageous, live for the moment and not be a good girl: nice, boring and blown up. What was the point? But this was not my parents' perspective. They had their own idea of what their Christian daughter should look like and let's say it was quite different from mine.

So the arguing started, and as fashion changed away from parallel trousers I wanted skintight ones that emphasized my developing hips. I humiliated Mum in shops and scorned her taste in public. I wanted to go to discos, not more meetings, and certainly not the ones my parents organized. That was my problem: my parents organized everything for Christian young people in Lisburn, except the discos that I was not allowed to go to. I was angry and enjoyed swearing, banging doors and shocking my loving parents by telling them to 'get a gun and put me out of my misery'. My brothers had always conformed, so this angry, rebellious female challenged everyone.

Somehow my faith got lost in my adolescence, as the child once so eager to help was replaced by a rebellious teenager who wanted to let everyone, including God, know that life did not make sense. My early gratitude was replaced by anger, as my links with God seemed to make life more difficult. Peer pressure made me want to blend in, not stand out. However, the fact was that I *was* different, because no one else's parents were sitting in the youth club foyer screening who came in, or planning the next youth church meetings, and the only places I could be anonymous were places where I wasn't allowed to be! Now that I was older and had attended many meetings, I had a deeper understanding of what it meant to follow God. I realized that it required self-discipline and the desire to live a holy life and produce the fruits of the Spirit.[2] Being sensitive, I could not cope with being rebellious *and* maintaining my faith. Somehow it felt easier to reject my Christian beliefs on the basis that they were my parents' beliefs, not mine.

After a while, things became more difficult when my dad

was made a Justice of the Peace. His qualities of fairness and honesty had been recognized, in addition to his able intellect, and so he was given additional responsibilities through which to serve his community. Being a quiet and unassuming man, Dad never boasted or spoke of his work and so I was unaware of the additional risks he was taking until my schoolfriend pointed them out: 'My dad was told to put extra security around our house, because he is a JP and the police told him that he may be in danger!' I went home and questioned my dad about this, but he passed it off in his usual modest way. 'God will look after us. I don't need to put extra security around our house,' he told me, and I wondered how he could trust that theory. People, including Christians, were being killed, maimed and scarred every day. Personally, I could not leave it to God.

I began to feel the need to protect our family and secretly decided to try to shield us all from sniper attack. Imagining members of the IRA trying to kill Dad or other family members, I initiated an evening ritual of making sure that after dark every door was shut in the house and every curtain closed, so that snipers could not see our whereabouts. My sleep became chequered with vivid dreams: running and hiding on our isolated roads, while being chased by terrorists.

Fear was reinforced again when, aged thirteen, I narrowly escaped injury at my father's business. One Saturday morning, after playing hockey at school, I arrived to get a lift home with Dad. I entered the front of the shop, passing through the household and paint departments before reaching the office to wait for him. While there, I heard a loud bang and realized that a bomb had gone off. There had been no warning. I saw panic in the faces of those around me as I ran towards the back exit, terrified of seeing my father or someone else I knew dismembered. Thankfully, it was not long before I heard that Dad had not been hurt.

However, others were not so fortunate: shrapnel from the explosion seriously injured three members of staff. Later it became apparent that a tin of paint had been returned to the shop with an incendiary device inside it.

When I was fifteen, I decided to end my rebellion. I was tired of being difficult and no longer wanted to fight continually with my parents. Actually I admired them and their unconditional love for me, and acknowledged that in recent years I had not earned it! I was reminded of the conversation I had had with Mum at my conversion, about how Jesus died for me even before I sought forgiveness for my wrongdoings,[3] and I wondered whether I should recommit my life to him. I gave myself an ultimatum: 'Live fully either for God or for yourself; don't live in between.' After some thought, I decided that I did have a Christian faith of my own, not just one borrowed from my parents. I did believe the Bible when it said that there is a loving Creator who wants a relationship with us.[4] So, aged fifteen, I made a public response to an altar call at a Billy Graham mission (though temporarily changed my mind when I saw how many of the counsellors were my parents' friends and happy to see me at the front for prayer. I baulked at the notion that I was now doing what lots of adults wanted me to do!).

Yet I was adult enough to see that rebellion for its own sake was pointless. It was better for me to live a life I believed in than not do something for the sake of being difficult. My return to faith gave me hope that God was able to make sense of life in Northern Ireland, as the endless atrocities still seemed completely pointless. However, in spite of them, I was now able to sleep better at night and adopt a more mature assessment of the situation. I realized that, compared with other areas, Lisburn was fairly safe and that the bombing of innocent people made terrorist groups unpopular. Also, I did not know of any JPs who had been murdered, so I shut out my alarming thoughts in the hope that I would never have to face them.

I was riding my bike with more balance now, as if my return to faith had given me an extra set of stabilizers, yet when I lifted up my head and looked ahead I still could not see where I was going. My future seemed bleak. I passed four O levels compared to my friends' eight or nine. I had no confidence in my ability to achieve, and could not imagine doing anything with success. The only thing I wanted to be was a nurse, but this too seemed out of my reach.

I returned to school to study English and domestic science A levels and resit English language and mathematics O levels. I hated school, especially after a teacher confirmed my fears of its academic élitism: 'Now we are left with the milk of the school,' she said. 'The cream – the rich and thick – have gone!' Having returned with minimum qualifications, I felt more like cream than milk, and this fear was confirmed in a careers interview, when the vice-principal told me to give up my dream of becoming a nurse as I was academically incapable. Since I knew I needed only one more O level to apply, I vowed to keep resitting my maths and English until I was successful. Within three months, I repeated and failed them again, but then resat them in June, six months later. However, I was miserable at school and plagued by physical symptoms of stress. I decided to leave at the end of the lower sixth without finishing my A levels, as I felt failure was inevitable one year later.

The following month I went on a residential youth Bible week with a group of friends, while waiting for my O level results. I had initially cancelled as I was feeling so stressed, but the leaders graciously allowed me to squeeze back in. The speaker explained that, not only did God want us to live a life according to Christian principles, but he also wanted to *use* our lives for his glory, if we yielded them to him. All we had to do was be willing to go wherever he sent us. For example, in the Old Testament, when God sent prophets to certain places, he also took care of the circumstances. When he sent Elijah to Mount Carmel, he honoured Elijah's obedience by performing a huge miracle,[5] setting fire to his sacrifice, even though it was doused with water.

I felt as though I had found a vital piece of a jigsaw: not only did I have to give my life to God and strive to live a holy life, but *he had plans for me*! I felt encouraged by the thought that all I had to do was go where he sent me and he would look after the circumstances. 'OK, Lord,' I prayed with renewed vigour and optimism. 'I will follow you. I will go wherever you send me and trust you to look after my life.' I returned home to discover a few days later that I had passed English language and maths at my third attempt! I was ecstatic; it felt like a miracle coming after year upon year of failure. I felt that at last God was opening some doors and giving me hope for the future.

Although still consumed by feelings of fear and inadequacy, I applied for nursing. Six months later, I moved to live in a nurses' home twenty miles away to start my training. I left the safety of my family, relieved that I had somehow survived my childhood route without the collision I had feared. Now God was leading me down a different road, and I travelled with childlike faith, confidently trusting that he would see me safely around the approaching hairpin bend.

3 A hidden dip

Just a quick glance beneath the surface of our life makes it clear that more is going on than loving God and loving others.

L. Crabb[1]

It felt like a sharp bend, because I could not envisage life beyond my first day as a trainee nurse. My elder brother drove me to the small cottage hospital in Newtownards, and we sat in silence listening to the radio as I considered my fate. I was completely terrified of every aspect of nursing, and, considering that I was still struggling to speak to men, the thought of carrying out intricate procedures in a male medical ward was shocking, to say the least!

My early days of training were excruciating as I coaxed myself to leave the sluice room and interact with patients. One Saturday evening, as I was feeding an elderly man a puréed meal of mince, and dodging the bits he spat back at me, I asked myself, 'What on earth am I doing here? It's Saturday night, I'm eighteen years old and I'm sitting in a hospital ward covered in regurgitated food!' Gradually the strain lessened as I adjusted to what was expected of me and began to care for my patients with more grace and with less of a puce face!

However, I found socializing away from home really difficult. I was not used to mixing with people who did not share my beliefs, and initially struggled to find the social skills I needed. During the first year, I could hardly eat anything in the canteen, as I was so nervous that I found it difficult to talk to colleagues and swallow food! However, over time, I made some very good friends and became more comfortable outside my home environment. Initially I did not find the academic side of nursing easy. I expected to fail as I had done at school, and consequently felt a lot of anxiety as exam deadlines approached. But I was surprised to discover that, when I did work, I *was* actually capable of passing!

Although the early days were traumatic, my faith carried me through. My belief that God was in overall control was a great comfort and helped me to ride the storms. Within six months I went down with severe flu, which meant I had to take some time off work and leave 'my crowd' of nurses and join a new group three months later. It was hard, but I was undeterred, as I believed with great certainty that God had enabled me to pass my O level resits so that I could embark on this career. So I did not focus on my feelings, but continued to cling to my belief that, whatever happened, God was in control of my circumstances.

Nursing was sobering: caring for people who were really suffering, and I coped by trying not to engage emotionally with their plight but by trying to relax outside work. There were lots of Christian social events to attend, including the Nurses' Christian Fellowship Bible study group. I was still unsure about how much I should engage in the secular world. After a couple of years, I moved out of the nurses' home and into a flat with other Christian nurses, where we had a great time together, supporting and encouraging one another. Increasingly, I believed that on completion of my training God would expect me to become a missionary and work abroad, using my skills where they were most needed, so I focused on preparing for that goal.

After three and a half years I qualified as a registered general nurse, and I started looking for a job as a staff nurse. I was unsuccessful in my own hospital as Tory staff cuts had hit our cottage hospital for the first time. Throughout my training I had spent a lot of time travelling, staying in Newtownards while I was working, and going back to my parents' house when I had time off. It felt as if I was continually moving between two destinations and belonging to neither. So when it came to looking for a permanent job, I decided to put down some roots. Since I was working towards living abroad as a missionary, I decided to apply for jobs in England and see how I managed being a bit further away from my family and friends.

When I boarded the Belfast–Liverpool boat, I knew that I was embarking on an adventure that placed me more on my own than ever before. I felt as if I had traded my bike, on which I was vulnerable and required lots of support, for a car with a chauffeur. I needed to be more robust, without the support of my family and friends, but would need to rely heavily on God, my driver, for direction. However, before long, I discovered that there was a hidden dip ahead.

I started working in a hospital in Dorchester, Dorset, in January 1985, as a newly qualified staff nurse on a surgical ward. Managing a ward was a bit of a nightmare for me because I soon discovered that time management was not my strength. Increasingly, I realized that the aspect of the job I was really interested in was talking to, and listening to, the patients. Unfortunately, this was the very thing I did not have time for. Often I would approach a task, reminding myself not to ask the person how he or she was feeling, because, if I did, I would become too involved in conversation and forget to give out medicines on time or send a colleague on her lunch break!

Also, I found it hard living in a new community. I felt like an outsider and was acutely aware that my accent was different. Months later, one friend told me that she thought there was something wrong with me, because I smiled so much at her when she was used to people ignoring her! I gravitated towards others who were more like me in background, and found myself spending more and more time with old friends from Northern Ireland who kindly took me under their wing. It was through them that I met a Christian girl called Denise, and within days of meeting each other we decided to look for accommodation together as we both needed to find something more permanent.

Under Denise's influence, my faith changed. When I met her, God was still quite a remote figure whom I was trying to please through service and holy living. While I believed he wanted to involve me in his plans, as he had done with people in the Bible, I did not expect these plans to take into account my personal desires. According to Denise, however, God was an intimate God, something demonstrated by Jesus, who spent his time helping ordinary people with their ordinary needs: assisting fishermen to catch fish and making sick people well, for example. 'We should ask for his help in the detail of our lives,' she said, 'and for us that means providing us with somewhere to live.' I was unsure about making such a specific request, but decided to give it a go. We drove down the A37 from Yeovil to Dorchester, praying that God would provide us with a place, preferably halfway along this twenty-mile stretch. We did not see anything remotely suitable, and I was less than optimistic that God was interested.

However, within a few days a member of staff at Denise's school offered us the most idyllic cottage we had ever seen.

It was in the heart of the Dorset hills, in a valley overlooking fields of grazing Jersey cows. It was remote, yet equidistant from both Yeovil and Dorchester.

Our prayer was answered and I began to feel that God was taking care of my new life. Here was a deeper fulfilment of the promise that, if I went where God sent me, he really *would* look after the consequences. Being away from friends and family was making me rely on God more, and I felt excited to see God leading me and providing for the details. I started to attend the same church as Denise, a fellowship church that was very different from my Presbyterian roots.

Although I was used to variety in worship through Mum and Dad's youth ministry, this new church still challenged me. It was much more emotional than I was used to. People became excited and often danced, clapped or waved their arms in a very enthusiastic way. Initially I was uncomfortable, and decided to ignore them by shutting my eyes and keeping control of myself, but as time went on I began to relax and allow God to speak to me through the emotional and spiritual energy. I enjoyed the fact that these people found faith exciting, as in recent years I had been finding mine hard work!

Life was busy, as I often started work at 7.30 am and finished late in the evening. But I wasn't someone who worried about rest. I had learnt through my childhood insomnia and nursing training that I could cope with little sleep. So I began to burn the candle at both ends, working hard and socializing. Both Denise and I enjoyed going out and having friends to stay. I was fortunate to have developed many good friendships over the years, through school, church groups and nursing. Many of my friends were a great support to me, and I valued and needed their ongoing contact.

During this time I had a brief relationship with a guy at church. Previously I had had only a few unpromising teenage encounters with boys. This was my first proper boyfriend and I liked him a lot, but felt scared of getting too involved because we were so different: he was so comfortable with himself and I was not. In the end, I broke off our relationship. However, I was gradually 'finding myself'. Since leaving Northern Ireland I had bought a denim jacket, got my ears pierced and had my hair highlighted. In a small community where everyone knew me I had found it hard to develop my own persona, but now, with anonymity, I was discovering who I felt comfortable being.

After a few months, I decided to apply for midwifery, and before long was accepted onto the course. I thought I was managing life well, so the early signs suggested that I would be able to cope if I lived and worked abroad. However, things were about to change. In September 1985, I developed a nasty flu-like infection. In my earnest, driven style I was reluctant to take time off work, so returned after only a week, still feeling very ill. Despite being told by my GP that I must rest, I fought the symptoms and continued to work despite experiencing nausea, muscle pain and weakness.

I left Dorchester Hospital at the end of October 1985 to start midwifery training, but soon afterwards went down with the same flu-like illness all over again. My first nine months of midwifery were plagued by sick leave, as my initial illness kept recurring.

Aside from this, I was not enjoying the training. I was twenty-two years old and still quite immature. I wasn't emotionally ready to empathize with my patients, and found them totally obsessed with themselves and their babies! But I believed that God would expect me to be willing to be a missionary abroad and, in order to be one, I needed midwifery. Although I did recover from my illness between relapses, it took weeks rather than days, and no sooner had I thrown myself into life again than I relapsed with the same symptoms.

Denise was adamant that God had not mapped out a miserable life for me: was it really his will for me to continue in a career I felt unable either to relate to or cope with? However, others at church were saying that they did not think that God would have opened the door to midwifery if he wanted me to shut it so soon.

Despite prayer, it was not clear what God wanted me to do, but ultimately I decided that I would leave. I was beginning to accept the fact that I did not actually want to become a missionary nurse, and felt unable to drive myself continually towards things that I felt I *ought* to do. I handed in my notice and felt vindicated when my Bible reading notes that evening suggested that sometimes God wants us to step out in faith without clear direction and make a new start.

In the ensuing weeks, I was torn between relief and fear. I could not live in England indefinitely without a job, but was at a complete loss as to what to do. I felt fed up with nursing and wanted something different. Although I had enjoyed certain aspects of the job, I had struggled increasingly. I recognized that I was struggling to be efficient and was more interested in the emotional, social and spiritual aspects of patients than their physical condition, something which often interfered with my ability to manage a ward!

The other issue was that Denise was moving to do her PGCE teacher training, and soon I would be without a flatmate. So in addition to needing a job, I also needed somewhere to live. I had limited resources, but decided to stay in England for as long as I could afford it. I decided to pray a very specific prayer to see whether God really did know and care about my needs. I felt as if God was urging me to do this and that he wanted to show me that he knew my thoughts from afar.[2] I was not just a Christian robot that he wanted to direct.

I was really sad that Denise was moving on but didn't have the energy to start again and live with others whom I did not know. I felt a deep need to have a place of my own, and I prayed too for a local job that I would like, as I could not face another move to a surrounding area. All this meant, I assumed, that I would take a break from nursing, as I could not imagine going back to our local hospital as a staff nurse and actually enjoying it. Consequently, I was not even considering jobs that involved nursing skills.

A few weeks later, as I scanned the local paper's employment section for jobs, I completely skipped over an advert for a school nurse in a local public school. That night I had a dream (the first and last of its kind) in which God told me that he wanted me to apply for that job. I woke up the next morning and looked at the advert more closely. I now felt differently about it and realized that, potentially, it was an answer to all my prayers: a flat of my own, as part of the package, adequate pay to stay on in England, and a satisfying means of using my nursing skills and my desire to support others emotionally and socially.

As I considered this post, I felt that God had used a dream to nudge me in a direction I would not have considered without his prompting. Maybe this was the evidence I was looking for, that God was interested in *me* and not just in my service to him?

Weeks later, I started the job and moved into the self-contained flat. The school was private with over 400 boarders and required three nurses to cover the sanatorium twenty-four hours a day, seven days a week during term time. It had a ten-bed unit for pupils suffering from anything from a stomach bug to chicken pox. The pupils ranged in age from eleven to eighteen and my job included running daily surgeries where they could drop in. I loved it, as much of the job required pastoral skills, and I felt known and valued by God. Now I really could entrust my life into his hands.

However, I was still not feeling very well physically. Five months after starting work, I contracted flu again, and this time I could not recover. I felt as though my new 'vehicle' was struggling to move. When I awoke each morning I had some energy to climb the stairs and carry out light duties. However, by lunchtime I would feel that my dial was flashing red, and by the evening I was unable to do anything; I was running on empty. The fact that this was ongoing frustrated and infuriated me.

I sought help from my church. Maybe God would heal me miraculously? I was starting to get used to the idea of signs and wonders and had every expectation that God would take this illness away from me. Regularly I sought prayer for healing, and forgiveness as I identified attitudes or behaviours that might be acting as a block to it. However, after months of confessing my sins and pleading for healing, I remained ill, and I wondered whether God wanted to teach me something through it. Some Christians around me were reluctant to accept this theory and became disenchanted when I started to refuse their offers of further prayer and counselling. Gradually, I withdrew from intense church involvement as I felt some people there were unable to accept me along with my illness. Their continual need to take 'victory' over it was actually making me feel worse.

After working at the school for one year, I suffered a major relapse. My temperature was high, and every muscle and joint ached. I could barely hold a cup of coffee. Whatever I had was getting worse, and I had to do something about it. Within a few weeks my parents arranged an appointment with a consultant neurologist in Northern Ireland. He listened carefully to my medical history and then told me that I had a post-viral illness, also known as ME (myalgic encephalomyelitis). He spoke in a very serious manner and told me that I was pushing my body too hard, and that it was vital that I stop work for six months or I might permanently damage my muscles and not be able to walk. He suggested that it would be at least two to three years before I would recover fully, and that in the meantime I would have to pace myself.

I could not believe my ears. I was twenty-four, single and sick. It now seemed as if I was going to give up work and live back at home with my mum and dad. I had not lived with them for seven years. Shame and disappointment enveloped me as I contemplated my diagnosis.

I needed to know more. I contacted the Myalgic Encephalomyelitis Association, but the news was not comforting. I read one story after another about people suffering crippling debilitation for anything from one to twenty years. When would my illness end, if ever? Where was God in all this? I was willing to serve him in any way he planned, but surely it was not his will for me to succumb to a debilitating illness and return to live a life of dependence? I felt angry, confused and hurt by certain Christians who made me feel guilty for having an illness that I despised and couldn't control, but deep down my faith in God was unwavering. He was directing my life and I was going to trust that he knew where he was leading me.

I never returned to my flat and had to let go of the many things I held dear: home, job, friends and health. Initially, I did not respond gracefully, but rather like a toddler lying on the floor screaming because things were not turning out as I had hoped. Yet nursing had shown me that things could be a lot worse, and I was grateful not to be suffering from a terminal illness.

Even after being back in Northern Ireland for some time, I felt anxious about Christians coming to visit in case they insisted on praying for me. However, my fears were unfounded, as all my friends and family were very sensitive to my spiritual needs and generous in their love to me. Since I was feeling too unwell to go to church anyway, I decided to meet God through writing journals and recording the details of my daily spiritual walk.

Through this, I learned to be more honest with God and see his provision for me in the intimate detail of life. It was as if I was shedding a layer of Christian politeness and really learning to communicate with him. Although I was suffering physically, I could still feel his presence, and writing my heartfelt thoughts drew us closer than ever before. It was as if my vehicle was stuck on a motorway in a hidden dip. I did not have the fuel to move forwards, so I sat waiting with God on the hard shoulder. My family and friends were very gracious to me, caring for me, taking me out, and listening to my fears without judging me. Yet I felt lonely. Without a job or good health, I longed for a partner to accompany and comfort me.

But meeting people was difficult and I felt that many men flipped their interest switch when they heard I was ill. During this period, I was fighting the pressure to believe that marriage partners can be found only after you have accepted singleness. In my suffering, I was honest enough to dismiss this view as unhelpful. I decided to keep an open mind and not put myself under the pressure of resigning myself to singleness.

After six months of rest and pacing myself at three-quarters of my energy levels (thus avoiding exhaustion), I started to look for opportunities within my limitations. Mum heard of a part-time job at my old school and I decided to apply. It was only ten hours a week for one term, and included manning the school sick bay and administering first aid. As it was the summer term it was very quiet, and I enjoyed entering the world of work again and finding something that I could cope with.

However, I found it challenging being back in my old school, and felt that God was exposing me to old wounds so that he could tend them and help them heal. Spending time in the school grounds reminded me of my feelings of worthlessness and hopelessness while a pupil there. Now, with nursing behind me, I realized how wrong this belief had been. I had proved that I had reasonable academic ability. I prayed for forgiveness for not having made the best of my education and asked for the ability to forgive my teachers and move on from their legacy.

Following that summer, I decided to study for an A level in sociology, with a view to going to university. I loved it and discovered that, although I had a lot of physical limitations, studying was something I could do at my own pace. I wrote out information on cards, which I stuck on the walls around my bed, so I felt that even when I was resting I was still learning. Life was slowly moving on again.

Driving to college to pick up my result, I discussed with a friend how possible it might be for me to fail this A level or not achieve the 'C' that I needed to get into Queen's University, Belfast to read psychology. After all, I had been studying sociology for only nine months. I had required extra time on medical grounds, and had had to push my body to keep going during exams. I had needed pain relief during the break and had had to lie down for thirty minutes. I had missed lots of lectures and had learnt only the minimum needed for the exams. Hence my incredulity when I opened the envelope and saw the grade I needed. 'I am going to university, me, the girl who failed at school and spent her whole time mucking about.' At last life was moving off the hard shoulder.

I was still suffering from post-viral symptoms, however, and needed to rest every afternoon, unable to do tasks on demand, but rather as energy allowed. I decided to move to Belfast so that I did not use all my energy travelling between Lisburn and university. Not having always been a model patient, I imagined my parents would breathe a sigh of relief. I had found it hard to be dependent in my mid-twenties and was often irritable, despite their support.

Providentially, a room came up in a house very close to the university. It was owned by some Christian friends and I enjoyed the opportunity to be independent again. My first year was chequered with exhaustion and stress as I tried to conquer four subjects, most of them brand new to me.

I began to attend a Presbyterian church and enjoyed the services. It was a good counterbalance for me after my charismatic church experience: open to the work of the Holy Spirit but also embracing a theology of suffering and social action, with church members actively involved in reconciliation within the province. I had a lot of respect for our minister and felt safe and inspired by his leadership. Over my first year at university my health gradually improved and, in spite of assignment extensions and shingles, I finished my first year successfully.

I completed my second year with even more ease and enjoyed the focus on my major subject, psychology. Now living outside Belfast, I was fit enough to study and travel within the same day. I was starting to look beyond my degree and wondered, since I enjoyed listening to people, whether I should train as a Christian counsellor. I started to read Christian psychology books and felt particularly drawn to and challenged by Larry Crabb's book *Inside Out*.

Crabb suggested that Christians often seem to try to avoid dealing with tensions in their own life by using the joy of their faith to *eliminate* or deny a painful experience rather than support them through it.[3] Often, inside their lives, there is more going on than loving God and loving others,[4] and sometimes their words or actions are born out of self-protection rather than genuine love: they are unable to recognize this subtle sin until they know what pain they seek protection from.[5] I was relieved to read such honesty, as my spirituality had been disturbing me for some time.

Certainly, when I had been ill, I had experienced pressure to use my faith to eliminate pain rather than support me through it, and I had never really worked this out in my mind. Also, I increasingly recognized that I was too concerned about creating the right image of myself rather than acting out of genuine emotion. For example, I rarely told anybody if they upset me, and did not like disagreeing with others, as I wanted to be liked and have friends.

I wanted to learn more about these ideas, and through research discovered that Larry Crabb had a seminary in Colorado, which taught his theories, leading to a Master of Arts in Biblical Counseling. This seemed perfect. I became excited at the prospect of taking this course, as it would enable me to train as a counsellor *and* face some uncomfortable personal issues at the same time. I decided to try to visit the United States over the summer and see whether this dream could become a reality. I discovered that there was a Christian conference centre close by and applied to work there as a summer student. However, when I contacted the centre, I was disappointed to discover that all their summer placements had already been allocated. It had all felt so right, and I had felt sure it was what God had wanted me to do.

It was after my second exam, when I was driving home, that I began thinking about Colorado again. I had a very strong feeling that God *was* going to make it possible for me to go there in the summer. I entered the house and hit the answering machine. I trembled with shock when I heard an American accent inviting me to go to work in Colorado in two weeks' time. A student had cancelled her placement and they now had one vacancy on the summer team. I leapt around the house like a crazy frog, ecstatic that God had opened this door for me and had even informed me in advance! I felt a renewed hope in my heart. Despite recent hardships, God still had plans for me.

Yet so many things were going through my mind: what if I relapse in Colorado? Will I be able to cope with the altitude? Will I cope with travelling so far on my own, especially as I don't like flying? A still, small voice quietened my soul and reminded me that it was all under God's control.

My second-year exams went well and I set off for America on a high. Recent memories of my monotonous life with ME seemed to be slipping away and I enjoyed the excitement of stepping out into something new and thrilling. I got out of the taxi and thought I had died and gone to heaven. Ravencrest Chalet was in the most beautiful location I had ever seen. This idyllic Christian holiday centre was at the top of a hill, overlooking the Colorado Rocky Mountain Range, and I gasped in awe at the dramatic scenery. All my disappointments seemed a million miles away.

It had been quite a journey to maturity, but I felt that my faith was now developing. I had experienced highs and lows in my walk with God, and was becoming ever more aware that I was not everything I wanted to be, and that, while loving God and loving others were my priorities, I was also living a self-protective life and at times 'managing' my image to appear better than I was. I had learned that God knew me intimately and could answer my personal prayers, but my ME had shown me that sometimes he did not answer as I expected. However, I felt at peace about that and able to co-operate with God in his plans for me, as he had given me strength to endure my suffering, and I had known the reassurance of his presence with me, even amid my loss and aloneness. I was now on a mountain top and felt that my hidden dip was completely out of sight.

4 Arriving at the precipice

Hope is the ability to listen to music of the future.
Faith is the courage to dance to it in the present.
Peter Kuzmic[1]

I spent the next few days exhausted because of the time change, and hyperventilating as my unfit body walked around the campus at an altitude of 8,000 feet. But I quickly adapted and began to enjoy the change in culture. I loved the openness of the people, even though it was a bit disconcerting at times. Conversations over lunch felt more like those I would have had at 2 am only with my closest friend, so I was challenged to become more open than usual. The beautiful scenery restored hope to my soul, and the disappointments of the previous years seemed to fall away.

The summer fled past as I worked hard, cleaning, preparing food, and serving regular, hazelnut and decaffeinated coffee. Before I knew it, my friend had arrived to join me in my last two weeks. We hired a car and drove cautiously around Colorado State with other international students on board.

Before I left the US I managed to fix up two interviews for Christian counselling courses, one in Larry Crabb's seminary and the other in Denver Seminary. While the lady at the first interview was pleasant, I found our meeting challenging: 'Why are you still single at twenty-eight? What about relationships? Do you relate well to men?' Suddenly I felt as if I was in a witness box. I felt uncomfortable – what had this got to do with my applying for the course? I had already realized in the previous three months that I found it harder than those around me to talk to strangers about my intimate feelings, and I feared that this would impede the subjective assessment process for this year-long Master's in Christian Counseling.

It was a different matter in the other seminary. A two-year course would not be financially viable unless I worked to support myself, and I could not imagine working as a nurse in America to support my theological training.

However, despite concerns about the courses, I returned home in the highest spirits following a fantastic summer, and declared myself recovered from my post-viral illness. Working hard at a high altitude had not induced a relapse, so I was obviously better. Free from the stigma of illness, I felt great. I was also seeing God lead me through a whole array of experiences, some difficult, but some wonderful. It was not always going to be hard. I felt optimistic and more able to entrust my future to God as I prayed, 'Lord, if you want me to go back to Colorado next year, let it happen. Keep my family well and protect me from anything that might stop me from leaving Ireland against your will.'

A few days later I met Steve at my friend's wedding. We had first met the previous year when I was a second-year student and working part-time in a Youth for Christ coffee shop. Initially I did not really consider him potential boyfriend material. He was younger than me, a postgraduate student who had never worked or lived outside Northern Ireland, and I assumed that I was too mature for him!

We had met for the odd cup of coffee and I had thought little of these encounters, but when Steve asked me to go to an Ulster Orchestra concert, I started to wonder what his intentions were. Following the concert, we went to a local restaurant. There I was surprised to discover that, despite our different lives, we related well to each other. After a few evenings out, I began to realize that I really did like him, and we began to spend a lot of time together. We already attended the same church and had many other things in common.

With Colorado still on the horizon, I busied myself with application forms and logistics while feeling very confused about why God had allowed someone so nice to enter my life at precisely the wrong time. Or was it? I had not gone looking for this, and in some ways had found love when I least wanted it. Throughout my illness I had been longing for a relationship, but now, when I did not have time for it, this lovely guy had come along. Could this be God's guidance?

At university the pressure was mounting as I completed two dissertations and prepared for my finals. I sat my American entrance exams and my results were sufficient to secure a place on the two-year postgraduate Christian counselling course. But how could I fund myself for two years? I knew that my savings would last for only one. Then I heard that the other college, which ran the one-year course, would consider my application only following my degree results, which would mean I would not be considered until a year after graduation! All this time, my relationship with Steve was steaming ahead. Struggling to manage all the variables, I decided to defer going to Colorado for a year and consider it again when my degree was finished.

After graduation, I slumped emotionally. Although I had achieved a good grade, it felt like an anticlimax. Getting into university had been a big deal for me, after years of academic failure, and I thought I would come out of it feeling all clever and confident. But I felt no different, and believed that I had merely been lucky in my exam questions. Steve was also feeling very low, as it was the first anniversary of his mother's death from breast cancer at the age of just forty-nine. We decided to go on holiday together despite our moods, to see how we got on. Much to our surprise, despite our emotional pain, we found an unexpected depth of companionship and comfort in each other's company. I began to believe that God had brought Steve into my life for a purpose. I read through my journals and found the prayer I had written asking God to protect me from anything that would stop me returning to Colorado. Since I had had only a few casual relationships in twenty-eight years, the fact that someone so special should come into my life now suggested this had come from God.

Three months later, Steve asked me to marry him, and we got engaged and married the following year, 1993. We were really fortunate to find a quirky, affordable house three miles from my hometown and eight miles from Belfast. Steve was now working for an aeronautical engineering company in Belfast as well as finishing his PhD, and I found a job as an unqualified residential social worker in a Christian rehabilitation centre in Belfast. Ever since I had been in Colorado, life had been manically busy: studying for the final year of my degree, meeting Steve, getting married, and now a new job. The belief triggered by Larry Crabb's book, that I needed to attend to my inner world, had long been pushed out.

My job, part of a project aimed at men with an alcohol addiction, was based in a challenging area of Belfast between staunch Catholic and Protestant areas. Although new to the area of addiction, I felt excited at being involved.

Within six weeks we had residents installed, and individual staff members took it in turns to sleep in the building.

It was such a joy to see men coming to the unit and regaining dignity and respect. For some, the opportunity to have a bath, shave and put on new clothes made them walk tall again within a few hours. My daily routine involved leading group discussions on topics such as sobriety, self-esteem and cognitive-behavioural patterns, which I had studied at university. I also gave out medicines, cooked meals, slept over, led counselling sessions, and did whatever else was required. A few months into my work, I decided to apply for formal social-work training, as I was very aware that I was leading groupwork and counselling without a relevant qualification. Following a group interview, I was accepted by Queen's University, Belfast for the Master's and Diploma in Social Work.

I had steep learning curves ahead at work before I started my course. Certainly the word 'naïve' described me aptly in the early days, but I soon got wise to men eating curries and disappearing in the early evening, and I learnt to detect those who were drinking alcohol on the premises and taking advantage of my good, if ill-informed, nature. Security was another learning curve. With minimal security measures – iron gates around the premises and iron bars on the windows – we, as staff, believed we were safe enough. However, while I was on honeymoon, a serious break-in occurred. Soon we had razor wire around the building, a telephone, a panic button and an intercom in the staff sleep-in room, and an internal alarm, which we set every night. It became our policy that, if the alarm went off during the night, staff were not allowed to leave their room but had to inform the police.

One normal evening I sat chatting to the residents and passively smoking their cigarettes until about 11 pm. I set the alarm, locked myself into my room and went to bed. A few hours later, I woke to the sound of the telephone ringing, and became conscious of the burglar alarm droning in the background. Disorientated from sleep, I answered the phone and heard one of the project's trustees telling me that the police had rung to tell him that the burglar alarm was going off. He asked me if I wanted him to come down. I said no, but I would ring the police, as our policy suggested. No sooner had I put the phone down than the police rang and I requested assistance to search the building. 'We do not want to send our officers into the area, madam, as it could be a set-up and therefore dangerous for them. You are based in a highly-charged sectarian area,' the policeman said.

'But I don't want to go and search the building on my own,' I pleaded. There was a pause. 'I will speak to my colleague and call you back.' I sat on the bed, shaking. It was as if I had suddenly woken up to how vulnerable I was.

One hour later, the police called to say they were outside. Nervously, I went downstairs and opened the front door. Two armed policemen greeted me. 'OK, madam, if you unlock all the doors in the area of the alarm, we will follow you.'

'Brilliant,' I thought to myself, 'so I get hit first and then you kill them!' We checked the area and all seemed fine. Half an hour later they left me to lock up and go back to bed. Weeks later, after my departure, I was told that a resident had confessed to setting off the alarm on purpose out of spite, as I had upset him in a group session that afternoon!

This experience took a lot out of me, and a meeting with a member of the management committee was arranged to discuss the incident. Shortly afterwards, two staff members were appointed for every sleep-in duty. The project went from strength to strength.

I enjoyed married life with Steve and found him very easy to live with. But one thing was niggling me: 'Are we doing enough for God?' My parents had had a joint ministry and I berated myself for not having one as well. In those early days of our marriage, I felt driven to find something

Steve and I could do together for God. We tried being youth leaders but both conceded that youth work was not our strong point. We prayed for God to lead us. I found it hard just to allow myself to enjoy our life together. Yet even within this anxiety to glorify God in our marriage I felt the hope of my faith: 'the ability to listen to the music of the future'. God had brought us together, and as long as we remained open to his leading, he had good plans for us[2] and would take care of our circumstances. However, it was not long before I had to exercise my faith and find 'courage to dance in the present' in the absence of music.

While I was in my second and final year of university, Steve was busy applying for other jobs. He had been unhappy at work, his position was insecure and, with the lack of suitable available jobs, we were willing to leave Northern Ireland, if that was what God wanted. At the same time, we stopped using contraception to see whether having a family was an option for us. I was thirty-two and had been told by my family planning clinic that it might be difficult for me to conceive, owing to the position of my womb. I had always realized that this could be a problem for anyone, so did not take too much notice of this warning, but equally I could not ignore it.

Therefore I was delighted, if a little shocked, to find out I was pregnant. It was our first month of trying, and everything had happened so easily. I was feeling well physically and was convinced that on my hospital visit in my twelfth week of pregnancy I would be reassured that everything was going smoothly. My friend Marion was with me, as Steve was away, and we were in good spirits. Marion was teasing me about the late-pregnancy waddle that lay ahead and we giggled as I lay awaiting a scan and the dreaded shock of the freezing KY jelly on my abdomen.

I was feeling pretty excited, and was planning to tell everyone our good news after this appointment. Then, after a time of prodding, I realized the nurse was struggling to find a heartbeat. 'I'll try a vaginal scan,' she said, and I shuddered as I got into an undignified position. 'This is a much more accurate scan; I am sure we will find it now,' she said. However, there was still no sign of life. Eventually, apologizing, she left to find a consultant. I had recently heard of a work colleague whose baby was dead in utero at twelve weeks, and I wondered if this was what was happening to me. Following another scan, I was told that there was no heartbeat and that my baby had probably died four weeks earlier. They would give me a week to adjust to the news and then would carry out one final scan before admitting me for an evacuation under general anaesthetic. On departure I rang Steve and cried down the phone, as Marion walked me to the car. I felt guilty that I had unwittingly involved her in our trauma.

Over the next week I was tortured by a whole range of emotions and coped with the horrific reality by using sturdy denial tactics. I took time off from my social-work placement and tried to keep busy at home, yet I could not escape the fact that I was carrying our dead baby. I longed to be taken into hospital for the operation I needed.

After what felt like an eternal week, Steve and I arrived at the hospital where our greatest fears were confirmed: our baby had died. I was duly taken to theatre to have it removed, and woke up crying as the reality hit me. Initially I was reassured that there were no complications, but two weeks later I was called back by the consultant, who told me that the laboratory had discovered an overgrowth of placental tissue. This meant I had had a hydatidiform mole, a rare complication of some unviable pregnancies, which would require subsequent regular check-ups as, very occasionally, if not fully removed, the tissue could become cancerous. I had been coping reasonably well until this latest news, but then I started to feel angry and frightened.

However, I was reassured that it was an easy condition to monitor, as it shows up in blood and urine tests, and that the worst part would be having monthly check-ups for at least a year, during which time I was not allowed to try for another baby.

A few weeks after this, Steve was offered a job in Bristol, one which he had applied for months before. 'Maybe this is all God's timing,' I said to Steve. 'If I was still pregnant I would not want to move away.' I knew that moving was unwise when you have just had a baby, as it increases the chance of post-natal depression. All in all, it seemed like a sensible time to move if we were going to take this step. Not trying for a baby for at least a year would give us some time to put down roots in a new community. Life was challenging and busy, so I did not notice how our strenuous journey was taking us towards a precarious edge.

It was a scorching day as we drove into Bristol, and neither of us knew exactly where we were going. I felt hot and bothered as I wove my way through the heavy traffic and maze of roads, trying not to lose Steve as we drove precariously in convoy. Eventually we found two parking spaces a short distance from our prospective flat. Steve went to collect the keys of our temporary accommodation, while I supervised the cars that were crammed with our worldly goods.

In the heat of the midday sun, I stood gazing at the elegant Georgian houses in front of me and felt a whole range of emotions. While I was excited about setting up a new home with Steve and exploring a new area and culture, I also felt immensely sad at leaving our home in Ireland. We had been very happy there, in our gorgeous, quirky seventeenth-century cottage near Belfast. Between us we had a large group of family and friends, and leaving them had been an enormous wrench.

Within a couple of days, Steve started work, and I felt more vulnerable than I had expected. Although our one-bedroomed flat was located in a lovely part of the city that was familiar to me, initially I felt very out of place and alone. Suddenly I had lots of time to myself, unlike in previous months, when I had been frantically saying goodbye to friends or working on my dissertation. Consequently, I had not had time to come to terms with recent events. The logistics of leaving, combined with the pressures of work, had totally preoccupied my mind, causing me to suppress all my feelings about our move and the recent miscarriage. My isolation and unease, together with the monthly sample boxes from Charing Cross Oncology Department, were constant reminders that all had not been well.

Soon we found a permanent dwelling in the area at a reasonable cost and we both started to feel that we were settling in our new location. After a few months I started working as a part-time social worker with older people and 'vulnerable adults'.[3] I also joined a gospel choir, a level-one British sign language class and a part-time Christian counselling course. Steve and I became housegroup leaders in our local church. Soon I was as busy as ever, with no time to stop and think.

During my counselling course, I was made to face recent hurts, and I sensed that my grief had been buried in an attempt to cope with the miscarriage. I had a series of six counselling sessions to discuss my sadness and then attended a Christian retreat in Cornwall to seek God and pray for healing. Here I came across a sculpture of a baby in its father's arms, and I had to buy it. I felt that this illustrated my belief that our child was in God's arms, and I wept as I drove back to show it to Steve in Bristol.

Six months after our arrival in Bristol, I was given the all-clear from the Oncology Department and told I could stop having monthly check-ups. This meant we could again proceed towards pregnancy. It was shortly after our first year in Bristol that I discovered I was pregnant again. I told myself, rather naïvely, that I had had my taste of hardship and that God owed me a break from trouble. (After all, I was a faithful servant!)

As a result, I approached my delivery date with a firm belief that God would make sure things progressed smoothly. I enjoyed the slower pace of life and the fact that I could no longer fly around doing umpteen things at once. I felt as if I was no longer travelling through life in a car but slowly hill-walking with Steve, accompanied by God as our guide.

The first indication of our ascent to the cliff edge was about six weeks before my baby arrived. I was told by my team manager, just before I left for maternity leave, that one of my clients' relatives had made an official complaint against me and my social-work practice.

The client suffered from Alzheimer's disease and was progressively losing her short-term memory. She had been quite a challenging patient and had often refused to allow professionals into her home. Once she had even stuck her tongue out at the psychiatrist from her living-room window, refusing to let him in. The following week I had taken her to the local hospital to see him as an outpatient.

Although this lady could not remember that I was a social worker, she did recognize me and would allow me to accompany her on these visits. I had to assist her regularly with tasks that were technically not part of my job. For example, I often took her to collect her pension or to buy some food at the local supermarket, as she refused to go with the plethora of home-care assistants who arrived to take her, having had so many that she could not remember who they were. Often on a Monday morning, I would get a report from the police to say that she had been found wandering round the neighbourhood at the weekend, unable to locate her house. So when she agreed to a trial period of residential care, everyone who knew her was delighted.

The only problem was that she was adamant that I should not contact her next of kin overseas to tell him of her decision. I sought advice from the psycho-geriatric consultant, who assessed her and said that she was still fit to make this decision. I knew that the Social Services Legal Department were bound by law to inform the next of kin within the trial period, so they would contact him within the next few weeks anyway. In addition, the woman's neighbours told me that they had informed her next of kin of the move already. I felt that my relationship with my client would be in jeopardy if I contacted him, so I decided to honour her wishes.

I knew this was a risky decision, as it involved a dilemma that social workers are familiar with: whose wishes do you aspire to respect, the client's or the relative's? Often in adult care they are at odds with each other. I considered telling the next of kin and then denying it to my client, but then, I thought, my personal integrity would be compromised.

When, two months later, my client's next of kin made a complaint against me, I was not totally surprised, but hoped that the three-stage investigation into my handling of the situation would uphold my professionalism. The first stage started immediately, with an in-depth interview by my team manager. I agreed for the procedure to continue while I was on maternity leave, as I felt fairly confident. I would be contacted again in due course if the complaint was carried to the second stage.

I had planned to take four weeks' maternity leave. I stuck the nursery border on the newly-painted walls and everything seemed to be going according to plan. The nursery was almost ready and we just had to organize the furniture. While I was feeling weary due to my advanced pregnancy, the complaint, and chronic concerns for my baby's well-being, I was also feeling hopeful of reaching our destination. I was about to become a mother and I enjoyed the nervous anticipation that entailed.

Unexpectedly, my waters burst and I went into labour three weeks early. Katherine was born safely two days later. It was as if we had finally reached the top of our precipice, the pinnacle of our dreams.

Since Colorado, life had been a mixture of experiences: the blessing and hope of family life with my husband, and the faith to believe in it despite the hardship and trauma of a complicated miscarriage. However, we now had a beautiful, healthy baby, and I looked away from the precipice, envisaging a smooth road down into happy family life.

* * *

5 Captive in rough terrain

The LORD hears the needy
and does not despise his captive people.
(Psalm 69:33)

'Why did I agree to that extra pain relief?' I cried anxiously
to Steve. 'If she dies now it will be my fault. I should never
have told the doctor she was in pain. She would be fine if he
had not given her the extra epidural.' Just at that moment a
nurse entered the room. 'We have some good news for you.
Katherine has been resuscitated. She was brought back to
life very quickly, so we are fairly confident that her brain has
not been damaged. Come in and see her now.'

I felt the chill of further shock, as these unexpected words
penetrated my soul. 'Katherine *has* been brought back to
life. She *is* going to survive!' I told myself, 'God has heard
our heartfelt cries; maybe he *does* know how much we can
bear?' Everything felt surreal and distant as if the nurse was
standing much further away from us than in reality: she had
spoken from the top of a precipice and now craned her neck
to see us amid the debris below.

We were led back into Katherine's ward where she was

again attached to lots of monitors, this time with her head encased in a transparent cube that released oxygen. Steve picked up a little knitted soldier and danced it around the box. Katherine followed it with her eyes, and her alertness told us that she had made a full recovery. I gazed at Steve and admired his ability to play at such a harrowing time.

The rest of the day was chequered with relief and fear, both for us and for the medical team. Immediately after Katherine's cardiac arrest, the anaesthetist made a full confession, saying that he had probably given her too much epidural top-up.[1] Then he spent the rest of the day retracting his story. I knew he was worried that we would sue him for damages, but we assured him that, on account of her swift recovery, we wouldn't dream of it. Maybe we would have felt differently if she had not survived?

Throughout Katherine's stay in hospital we barely left her side. I felt particularly jumpy and anxious, finding the sound of monitor alarms terrifying. I now knew what it would be like to lose Katherine and did not ever want to go through that experience again. Katherine meant so much to me, and the thought of losing her was unbearable. Anxiety started to dictate: 'You need to look out for her, even more than before. It is up to you. Look, you cannot even trust the hospital to care for her. Even *God* nearly let her go. You can't trust anyone. If you had gone for breakfast on Monday morning, Katherine would have died. She didn't have any monitors on and the nurse wasn't with her when she stopped breathing. No, it was your instinct that kept you there. Katherine's survival depends on you!'

Following a good recovery, Katherine was discharged from hospital five days later. Assisting us to the car, a nurse beamed and instructed us to 'take her home and enjoy her'. I stared back, incredulous. I felt so afraid of the future. If the past was anything to go by, life was very dangerous. I needed to stay vigilant and be prepared to fend off future disasters. How could the nurse expect us to enjoy life when it was so fragile?

Returning home was not easy for me, but Steve appeared to be more relaxed. He focused on the miracle of the last few days: how we had remained with Katherine during her critical hour. Although I could acknowledge the miracle, I still felt traumatized and distressed by the memory of almost losing her. It was as if Steve had quickly recovered from our fall, dusted himself down and started to enjoy full mobility, whereas I was shattered and immobilized.

In addition to the trauma, I was still adapting to motherhood. I had been completely unprepared for it, as I had had minimal experience with children or babies until now. Three months on, I was aware more than ever that my life had changed for good. While I welcomed the changes, I was also challenged by them: struggling with the loss of time to myself and desperate for sleep and for space to recover from our trauma. I missed simple things such as being able to walk to the corner shop on my own and have time to process my thoughts. Yet, at the same time, everything beyond Katherine seemed pushed to the backstage of life: work and personal leisure seemed vaguely distant, irrelevant memories, meaningless compared with the importance of her survival.

Sensing my difficulties, my mum flew over from Ireland for a few days to support us. It was such a comfort to have her with me. I began to believe that things were going to settle down, but then the next set of events started to unfold.

Shortly after Mum's departure, I received a telephone call from another Social Services team manager, whom I had never met, asking if she could come and interview me as part of the ongoing complaints procedure. First of all, she asked me about the most recent allegations made two months earlier, when Katherine was two weeks old, that I had stolen from this client. I strongly refuted this, but felt vulnerable, as I knew this client could not vouch for me because of her memory loss. The manager conducted the interview in a formal manner, asking me detailed questions and recording my answers diligently. She said that she would inform me of her verdict in due course. I had been through so much recently, and Katherine was all that mattered to me now. Social Services could even fire me if they liked; I was too worn out to fret.

Then, on a Sunday morning ten days after discharge, Katherine started to cry a lot more. I became really anxious, as I felt this was unusual for post-operative recovery and indicated a complication. Steve was cooking lunch and I berated him for attending to food at such a time. I rang the staff at Accident and Emergency to discuss this development and they summoned us immediately. They checked Katherine over and said that they could not find any reason for her crying, and that some discomfort was to be expected. However, they reminded us that she had had a very serious operation and that we should monitor her carefully and return if we had any further concerns. She would be reviewed again in three weeks' time. The words 'very serious' reverberated around my head as I reminded myself yet again that Katherine's survival was now largely down to me, as Steve had returned to work. I could not afford to relax for one minute.

A few days later, I met some mums and their babies for a picnic. Our first four months had been so different from theirs and I resented hearing about their offsprings' steady progress: one baby had been sleeping through the night since he was seven weeks old, and all the mums described their increasing adjustment to their new status. I, on the other hand, still felt 'all over the show' and had not yet developed any routine. During the afternoon, tears poured down my face as Katherine pulled off my breast and screamed when I tried to feed her. I explained that she was crying a lot during breastfeeding and that I was worried I was not producing enough milk to satisfy her. The mums listened sympathetically and suggested that I should seek professional advice, as none of their babies had ever fed like that. I left the picnic feeling humiliated, as they seemed to have a clearer perspective on feeding my baby than I had. Katherine's crying had become normal to me.

I duly went to see my GP, who suggested that I stop breastfeeding Katherine and try feeding her formula milk from a bottle. He thought it was possible that my milk production was insufficient and had been adversely affected by our circumstances. Steve and I agreed that it was worth trying, as we were all becoming upset around feeding times. However, I felt angry at having to give up breastfeeding, as I had always planned to breastfeed Katherine for much longer, believing that it was the best thing for her. I felt I was being robbed of another vital aspect of early motherhood.

Shortly after I stopped breastfeeding, we made an amazing discovery: Katherine would feed really well in the morning (taking a full bottle), but, as the day progressed, she would refuse milk, drinking less and less until she barely fed at all. We made an immediate appointment with the hospital Outpatients' Department, where the registrar told us that this was probably owing to oesophageal reflux, which was to be expected after her type of operation! 'Thanks for *not* warning me,' I moaned to myself. 'Katherine has had to endure yet another round of needless pain!' In Outpatients she was prescribed two drugs, and so we entered the world of infant medication. One drug was to be drawn up in a syringe and squirted into her mouth half an hour before every feed, to help empty her stomach and make room for the next feed, and the other had to be added to her bottles.

More stuff to think about. Why could things not be easy, as they were for others? I longed for Katherine's pain to go away and for our lives to be free from fear.

In the early afternoon, I duly drew up Katherine's first dose of medication, as instructed. Steve checked it too and we gave it to her without much thought. Our housegroup were coming round for a meal that evening, so we were busy preparing for their arrival. Then Katherine started to cry even more than in recent days. 'What on earth is going on?' I asked myself. 'Things are getting even worse. Can this be normal?' We tried to manage by nursing Katherine and dismissing our fears until the time came to give her another dose of medication. I felt that her reaction to the initial dose was unnatural.

Finally, at 5.30 pm, before we gave her a second dose, we succumbed to our concerns and decided to ring our GP and ask him if it was possible that the medication could cause stomach pain. He confirmed that this could be a side effect, so I immediately rang the hospital and spoke to a registrar. She quizzed me on Katherine's weight and the dose and then informed me that one of the drugs had been prescribed at the wrong dosage! We were giving her two and half times more than she should have been receiving at her weight, which explained her acute abdominal pain! I was furious, and made a mental note never to see a registrar again in Outpatients. We would see only the most experienced doctors from now on! Yet again the message was becoming clear to me: 'Life is dangerous; life is unstable, and it's up to you, Hazel, as the primary caregiver, to make sure that your daughter survives!' Not being someone who paid a lot of attention to my emotional world, I tried to concentrate solely on my baby's health, until my internal turmoil found a way of catching my attention!

First of all it was insidious. I became aware of increasingly negative thoughts and feelings about myself: 'I have failed as a mother. Other parents don't make mistakes like I do. I have allowed my daughter to suffer needlessly. I knew something was wrong, so why didn't I do more about it?' I found it difficult to come to terms with the fact that I had dismissed my instinctive sense that there *was* something physically wrong with Katherine in favour of the advice of the professionals. This made me angry with myself. However, the other voice saying that I had facilitated Katherine's survival was inaudible.

Negativity seemed to run up from behind and overwhelm me. Before I knew it, I had moved from having some guilty feelings to a state of self-loathing and hatred. 'I have let Katherine and Steve down. I am not worthy to be a mother. I am worse than all the others. They would be much better off without me. Take an overdose, take an overdose. I still have the antidepressants that the doctor prescribed for me a few months ago. What would happen if I took them all? Would they kill me or would I survive in a vegetative state? Katherine won't miss me, as she hardly knows me. She won't remember me if I go now. Steve can meet a more capable wife. They will both be better off without me.'

I felt very confused and afraid. Things had never been this serious before. I had previously taken pride in my ability to deal with anxiety and focus on positive thoughts amidst adversity, but nothing was clear any more and I feared that I would actually succumb to these negative voices. I could not rationalize them, or control their frequency. I felt as if a huge magnet had been inserted into my head, which was now being pulled down by a negative force into a chaotic and rough place. I was marooned and powerless; the darkest of thoughts just ran amok throughout my mind. I felt mentally broken, as if I was crawling in rough terrain with my head bumping along the ground, bleeding and bruised, and I was unable to lift it up. Steve and Katherine seemed to be trying to rescue me from afar.

Then, despite being at rock bottom, I started to feel even worse. I developed extreme feelings of terror and agitation as I began to become obsessive about my fears. It's bad enough having lots of negative thoughts and feelings, but, in my experience, when one negative thought becomes constant and repetitive, in conjunction with a very low mood, life becomes unbearable. It was as if I was stuck in a corner where a negative force kept repeatedly banging my head against the same rock, until my captors arrived.

To begin with, I thought I was just being silly when I found myself constantly worrying about the trivial matter of whether or not Katherine was smiling at *me*. I believed she was smiling at others, but withholding her positive response from me. 'Maybe she does not like my glasses, or my face is somehow unpleasant to her,' I mused to myself. 'Maybe she can see something in me that she doesn't like.' Strangely, at one level, I recognized that this thought was ridiculous, and could acknowledge that Katherine had been smiling at me normally for most of her life (and, understandably, she did not smile at anyone when she was in pain). Despite this awareness, I was totally consumed with the same thought and experienced a fearful adrenalin rush every time it came to mind. Yet, as soon as Katherine smiled at me, I had to start all over again to seek the next positive response, and the next and the next. I had never experienced anything like this and realized that mentally I was in deep trouble. Incredulous, I could not accept that, at this most important time in my life, I was falling apart.

I had always believed that I would rise to any occasion and that God would give me the strength to do so. Yet it was as if my mind had become an armed captor and was holding me hostage, with a gun to my head, replaying the same lines from a scratched record, saying, 'Listen to me or lose your life!' Alongside my captor's taunts, my inability to think through his threats made me feel as if I was surrounded by a thick fog, which obliterated my perspective on the situation. I recognized that I was in desperate need of help.

Terrified and bewildered, I sat in the doctor's surgery and described my mental mayhem. The doctor listened attentively, smiling reassuringly as I talked. This surprised me, as she did not seem alarmed by my symptoms. 'Surely she hasn't heard this before? There can't be many others who have felt like this,' I thought. After listening to me for a while, my GP said that she believed I was now suffering from post-natal depression. I could not believe that post-natal depression felt like this. Surely I was feeling too awful to be just *depressed*? I thought depression was merely a gloomy feeling, not at all like the crippling sadness, loss of reality and terror that I was experiencing. I explained that I still had antidepressants from my previous prescription which I had not taken, and she suggested that I should start taking them immediately. I agreed, but left her office terrified, dreading what fate would befall me now. 'What if the tablets make me feel even *worse*?' However, stuck between a rock and a hard place, I just had to try them.

I was distraught because I felt that the mere presence of my obsessional anxieties proved that I was unworthy of parenthood: evidence that I was not good enough to be Katherine's mother. Yet the more I tried to rationalize them, the more they returned with a vengeance. 'Katherine is rejecting you. Look, she smiles at Steve and perfect strangers, but not at you. You've screwed up, and even at six months she knows that. You do not deserve her. She is withholding her response to you in protest.' I felt as if these messages were being relayed to me through a negotiator, and my ransom was to show that Katherine did respond to me and that I was a worthy mother. All this reinforced my compulsion to check that these thoughts were wrong and compile evidence to the contrary, but my brokenness precluded this. It was as if my memory was not working, as I could not remember previous responses in order to refute these accusations. I felt mentally confused and chaotic, and everything I did was underpinned by this reality. Nothing else mattered except securing release from my captors.

I started immediately on a low dose of Prothiaden, also known as Dothiepin, and gradually increased it during my first week. It belongs to the tricyclic group of antidepressants, being one of the 'older' tablets. (It had been prescribed earlier because I was still breastfeeding at the time and my doctor had told me it was unlikely to affect Katherine.) I felt terrified as I took my first capsule, not really knowing what to expect. The thought of taking anything that might alter my mood was petrifying, as I felt that, if I made one wrong move, my captor might blow my head off. If I did anything that would make me feel worse, I might succumb to the depressive thoughts that advocated peace of mind by taking an overdose.

After taking my prescribed dose for a week, I returned to see my doctor for a progress review. I appreciated her empathy – I could see in her face that she was concerned for me. I told her that we were about to go on holiday to a cottage in Devon and I felt very nervous about leaving the security of my home and its close proximity to the surgery. She seemed to understand my acute vulnerability and said I could ring her from Devon if I needed to. I was moved by her thoughtfulness and felt as if she had thrown me a rope and attached me in a secure position, reassuring me that, if I moved, my rough terrain would not crumble and consume me and that I would not fall further into the darkness alone.

A couple of friends came to join us in what was to be our first holiday with Katherine, apart from visits to family in Ireland. I felt very agitated and upset and found it hard to accept the direction my life was taking. I had so much wanted to be a perfect mother, successful in everything I did, and I could not accept my 'illness'. I felt so sad that I could not enjoy Devon or focus on its natural beauty, as all I wanted was to know the answer to my questions: would the tablets work? How long would they take, and was I damaging my relationship with Katherine by becoming depressed or taking medication? I began to realize that waiting for medication to work is a very frightening time. Although I had taken a step forward when I had found the courage to acknowledge that I was ill and started treatment, I now felt as if I had moved backwards, as I dealt with the added worry of whether the medication was going to make me feel better or worse.

Steve and I coped with our week away by trying to survive each moment and minimize the impact of my depression on Katherine as much as possible. Having a diagnosis at least enabled me to understand that something outside my control was happening to me, and, terrifying though this was, I conceded that I could not help it. I tried to strike a balance between spending time with others and taking the opportunity to rest. The relentlessness of my anxieties was exhausting, and this week offered me the chance to get some extra sleep.

I was surrounded by so many things that ordinarily would have filled me with joy and hope: a beautiful baby whom I adored, my supportive husband and friends whom I loved, and a beautiful cottage in an idyllic location. My sadness affected everything, and I found even small tasks difficult. For example, I dreaded changing Katherine's nappy as I had to look her straight in the face, and I felt so low that I found it hard to think of anything funny or cheerful to say to her. It was then that I discovered that if I put on music (nursery rhymes or silly songs), I was able to rise above my anxieties and smile quite naturally. And so this previously difficult task became enjoyable, and I began to recognize that, even within severe post-natal depression, happy moments can be created and savoured.

Thankfully, a few weeks later, my medication gave me some distance from my terrifying thoughts and feelings. I welcomed the dulling of my fears and gradually noticed less need to check Katherine's facial responses. It was as if my captor had taken his gun out of my face and placed it down by his side. He would raise it from time to time in intimidation, but mostly it lay there as I listened to his accusatory mutterings. I still felt impaired by foggy thinking, as, in addition to my mental fragility, the medication slowed down my cognitive processes. Although the thought of checking Katherine's facial response to me was still present, the compulsion to do so gradually waned.

As soon as I stabilized, I booked some private counselling sessions to give me the opportunity to talk about the trauma, in the hope that this would release some pressure and improve my mental health. I was fortunate to know a professional counsellor through my Christian counselling course, so in many ways it felt as if I was letting off steam to a friend rather than receiving 'therapy'.

During these sessions I was not fit to stand back from the situation and analyse it, as it was still too challenging. But they met my desperate need to talk and cry about my terror of losing Katherine. Having a counsellor who was a Christian helped, as I was also able to touch on feelings that were linked to my faith: how I felt let down by God because he had allowed Katherine's cardiac arrest. Through talking, I was able to see more clearly that God *had* in fact answered my greatest plea, for Katherine's survival, although my deepest questions remained: why did God allow me to fall into the trap of depression at such a crucial time in my life, and would he get me out of it? Using a non-directive approach, my counsellor supported me while I found my own answers, rather than directing me to specific solutions.

I left this series of sessions with a greater clarity, but still without all the answers.

Over the next few months, the overwhelming sadness and acute anxiety gradually eased. Since the complaint procedure from work was still ongoing, I decided not to return to my old job. Shortly after the team manager had interviewed me at home, I received a letter from her saying that she could find no evidence of professional negligence or malpractice. However, the complainant had chosen to challenge this outcome and take the complaint to the third stage: a hearing in front of a panel. I found the whole procedure very stressful, particularly when I had enough of my own personal worries to contend with. Consequently, I decided I would not go back to social work until my life had stabilized and I could cope with the possibility of another client or relative making a complaint against me. In the meantime, I applied to work for a family I had met through antenatal classes. James, a wheelchair user, required a personal assistant to help him look after his baby daughter while his wife was at work. I started in January 1998 when Katherine was seven months old, and we all got on very well together.

A few months later, the police visited my home to interview me regarding the allegations of stealing money and acting suspiciously in the client's house. It was a horrible experience and I felt as if I were being treated as 'guilty until proven innocent' and, because of my client's memory loss, she could not support me in refuting the allegations. However, due to a total lack of evidence, the case was dropped. A short time afterwards the complaints panel met and decided in my favour: they did not uphold the complaint. Another nasty experience was put behind me.

Six months after starting work for James and his family, I started to feel well enough to come off medication. Steve and I discussed it and agreed that we would like to have another baby, sooner rather than later. I had already started to plan my next pregnancy when my GP warned me to not get pregnant again too quickly, as research indicates that women who have their children very close together are more likely to develop post-natal depression. But she conceded that I could start reducing my medication slowly, with a view to preparing for pregnancy. Within three months, I had reduced my medication to half, and then the trouble started. It was as though I had fallen into a deep pit close to the exit to my wild place. While I believed my captor had left the jungle, I soon discovered he had merely gone for reinforcements!

Grateful to God for answering our prayers for Katherine but still bemused by my acute anxiety and depression, I hoped that God was going to demonstrate his support for me in the place of captivity by securing my imminent release. But my faith was about to be further tested, as I relapsed instead into a deeper state of anxiety and depression.

6 Meeting Despair

The Imp of the Perverse will try to torment you with thoughts of whatever it is you consider to be the most inappropriate or awful thing that you could do.
Lee Baer[1]

Completely out of the blue, a disconcerting question went through my mind, forcing my self-confidence out of me as if rammed by the impact of my fall. Lying in a deep, dark crater and feeling entangled in a haze of anxious thoughts, I asked myself, 'How do I know I am good enough to be Katherine's parent? How do I know I am not really a paedophile or a child abuser?'

Now that I am well, I can immediately think of numerous robust answers refuting this thought, but then, in a foggy and sedated stupor, I could not think it through, and the ensuing fear precluded all chance of rational thought. It was as if in my depression I had developed an extreme awareness and fear of my human frailty and completely lost my previous sense of God's love for me and of being created in his image.

Numerous armed recruits surrounded my dark place and

laughed at the thought that I should escape so easily. They demanded immediate evidence to disprove their sordid accusations and threatened to remove me permanently from my husband and daughter if I could not provide it. Ensnared, I felt totally overwhelmed and alone.

Clever enough to remind me that I had met convicted paedophiles through my social-work practice, my interrogators brought to mind their faces and the fact that they looked and behaved normally. I needed stronger evidence than mere external reassurance, as I knew that those capable of these crimes had agendas that were hidden even from their nearest and dearest. So words of comfort from my disconcerted husband were unable to help me as I moved towards a living hell on earth, for losing faith in myself opened up the possibility of my being capable of anything, casting doubt on the very person I had believed myself to be.

I was horrified at the mere hint that I should be capable of such a crime and felt tremendously guilty that it should even enter my head. However, what was more worrying was that I had not immediately been able to dismiss the idea with confidence. Insidiously, my thoughts asked, 'How do you *know*? Surely the fact that you are worried is evidence that you are capable of this crime. Don't they say there is no smoke without fire?'

If I had been obsessed before, I was triply obsessed now. I needed to know the answer for sure, and wondered whether I should pack my bag and leave our family home while I figured it all out. 'How could my life be reduced to this?' I wondered. 'I have a beautiful daughter and I am scared to be with her.' I found myself analysing how long it took me to change a nappy and asking myself if I was taking too long. Was I staring in places where I should not stare? Were these thoughts evidence that I was an inappropriate mother? Broken, desperate and ashamed, I returned to my

GP and blurted out my fears in a torrent of tears, willing to face the consequences of my confessions. Through the blur of watery eyes, I noticed that she was still looking at me sympathetically. She said she thought my depression was coming back and that I might need new medication. She would make an urgent referral to a psychiatrist for some expert advice, and in the meantime I needed to continue to take the reduced dose.

The next three weeks were terrifying, as I waited for my appointment. I felt petrified that the psychiatrist would be unable to help me, leaving me to manage my symptoms alone, and I felt I could not go on like this for much longer. Somehow I forced myself to continue with my normal routine and attend to Katherine's needs while managing the damning personal accusations and constant scrutiny of my internal world. I dreaded having to share my terrifying and humiliating thoughts with a complete stranger, especially a psychiatrist! 'What if he/she believes my fears? How can I convince someone of my innocence when I doubt it myself? Maybe I will be admitted to hospital or maybe they will take Katherine away. I could not bear to live without her.'

Desperate, I decided to ask for prayer, as I felt the only way I was going to get through the next few weeks was by a miracle. Unsure whom I could trust with the contents of my troubled mind, I decided to ring a mum from church who was involved in the pastoral care of families. I rang and explained briefly that I was really struggling, and asked if she would meet to pray with me as soon as possible. She kindly agreed, but when she said that it would be 'cool', I wondered whether she was really going to understand my desperation. We duly met within a few days.

When I arrived at her house, I was feeling optimistic that this was going to be my day of healing. 'Maybe God wants to show me that he, and not the psychiatrist, is the real healer.' I was excited at the prospect of such a testimony:

'Tormented and afraid, I prayed, and God took away my fears. I threw away my medication and never looked back!' I marvelled at the idea and hoped that God was going to use my desperation to give glory to himself.

During my visit, I found it easy to speak openly about my situation, as I felt confident that I was sharing with someone who would vouch for my integrity. However, as I spoke, I felt increasingly that my listener was (perhaps understandably) uncomfortable with the nature of my worries, and that she managed our time together in a formal, distant manner. Despite this, we persisted in prayer, and I left feeling that I had fulfilled my responsibility to God, humbly laying my requests before him.[2] At the same time, I felt that this meeting had proved to me that my burden was too heavy for others to bear and that I would experience only further hurt if I shared it outside my marital walls. This was confirmed when my 'prayer partner' never again asked me how I was or referred to our conversation!

However, the following day I woke up feeling hopeful that God might have healed me. But it was not long before I was back into circular thinking, checking myself as I changed a nappy and bathed Katherine. So I was grateful when the day eventually arrived for me to go to the Psychiatric Outpatients Department and share my relentless fears.

It was bad enough to have to go at all, without having another person to witness my degradation, so when Steve came home from work early to look after Katherine, I left with only the company of my cerebral tormentors. The clinic was not far from our house and I walked the mile in nervous trepidation. On arrival, confronted with the buzzer at reception, I suddenly felt embarrassed as I publicly declared my name and consequently my need for psychiatric help. The door opened and I made my entry. The building felt dark and dismal as I gave my appointment details to the receptionist. I was relieved that I did not meet anyone I knew in the corridor, and hoped ex-clients would not greet me in the waiting room.

Dog-eared glossy magazines lay on a corner table in the small waiting area, which had grubby walls covered with self-help posters. My stomach churned with terror as I reminded myself of what lay ahead. Normally I was the helper, the social worker, and I entered these places in support of others, but now it was I who needed help, and I hated this development. Two people were seated already, and I scrutinized them for signs of insanity. Would I become like them? Should I be more worried than I already was? Relief and nausea arrived in tandem as my name was called just moments after my arrival.

The doctor, who looked younger than me, ushered me into a nearby side room. I wondered just how much he would understand my torment. However, he quickly impressed me with his mature approach, recognizing my immediate need to talk about my turmoil as I made a full confession of my thoughts and fears. Desperate for reassurance, I needed to share the responsibility with others. Maybe he could help me see if I was a fit mother, or whether I should leave the family home.

Shoulders bent, leaning towards me, and speaking in a quiet voice, he looked straight into my eyes and said, 'I don't think you would hurt your baby and I am sure you are a good mother. I think your depression has come back because you have reduced your tablets too soon, and these fears are the symptoms. I have heard other mothers say similar things; you are not the only person to worry about this kind of thing.'

His words helped, but due to my dark place, they brought only very temporary relief. 'How does he know what I am capable of? We have just met, so I can't really take reassurance from his words, can I?' He suggested that I should return immediately to my original dose of medication because it had previously given me some respite from my worries, explaining that the dose I was currently taking was not a therapeutic dose.[3] I began to understand why my worrying had returned, though I still wondered deep down whether the reduction in medication was the real reason for these thoughts or whether they were due to my malign character.

Walking down the hill towards home, I felt totally alone as I went over the conversation with the doctor in my mind. I just couldn't believe that my life was reduced to sitting in a psychiatrist's office, seeking validation of my thoughts from a complete stranger, and even he could not give me what I needed: confidence that I was who I thought I was, and not who I feared I was.

Broken, desperate and humiliated, I entered the house. When I saw Katherine and Steve, my heart felt like it was going to explode in agony for them. They did not deserve this madness in their lives and I felt *so* ashamed that I was the cause of it. They greeted me with their usual loving responses, which reminded me that life was worth living after all, despite its anguish. I was so lucky to have these two people to come home to – what would I do without them?

Steve was keen to hear about my visit, and I longed to give him the instant reassurance and solution that we both yearned for. Yet I felt I had little to say except that the doctor had suggested I increase my medication again and 'hoped' that the tablets would work second time round, and that my symptoms had been due to their reduction. I found it humiliating and utterly unbearable to have to tell him of these worries and trawl through my fractured mental processes. I longed to be the person I had been before. How I hated the person I had become! Steve listened and I sensed his anxiety and bewilderment, as, like me, up to a few weeks earlier he had thought things were getting better and that we were moving on towards our dream of having a sibling for Katherine.

Later that evening, as I sat in the living room while Steve read Katherine a bedtime story, I felt at my lowest point. I listened to a new voice of torment, as another, senior, officer spoke more loudly and distinctively. His words particularly penetrated my being. This was Despair, Major Despair.

'There is evidence that you are not turning out to be the person we expected you to be. For example, others have seen ill in you and cast suspicion on your character: you have been the subject of a professional inquiry in which caring relatives and neighbours thought you were capable of stealing and abusing the trust of a vulnerable adult. Also, I believe that in the past you have been slow to represent your daughter's needs, that you missed her illness and allowed her to suffer needlessly. This is not good enough and I wonder what else you are capable of?'

'Interesting,' he said scathingly, 'that you have developed these sinister thoughts. I wonder whether this implies a darker side of your personality that is waiting to emerge. You have even sought help from your God, yet he withholds his help, and his people are wary of you.'

'You will stay imprisoned and under constant scrutiny until you provide me with 100% proof that these accusations are untrue. However, refuting these allegations is not enough. I need to know with certainty that your self-doubt does not indicate a potential threat. Remember, this situation is affecting not only your own life, but the lives of your child and your husband. The more quickly you provide evidence, the more quickly you will be released.'

Despair's arguments seemed so plausible in the dark, murky atmosphere of the harsh environment. I could not see anything clearly except that it was up to me to get myself out and that nobody else seemed able to rescue me. I knew I had *not* committed an unlawful act, but had no idea how to prove to myself or anyone else that I would not commit a crime in future. Desperate, I looked towards Major

Despair as he suggested I end my life and enter a peaceful oblivion. 'Surely it would be sweeter?' he whispered. A deadly darkness enveloped me, as if the sky had been emptied of all light.

'No matter how bad things get, *I will not give up*,' I retorted. 'I know I am not a threat to my daughter, and I am *not* going to let you ruin my family's life. I will overcome you and your cruel army; I just don't know how to do it at this moment.' Despair refused to leave, causing his formidable shadow to hang over me, but I reminded myself that any voice that taunts you, tempting you to end your life, is not from God and *not* safe to follow, and although I could not stop Despair's speech, I vowed to oppose it until it fell silent.

I had been through too much to succumb to the lure of Despair and, although I yearned for relief from my mental torture, I did not want it at any cost. My belief in God had become too real to give it up now and take things into my own hands. I was fortunate that I had seen God at work in my life already, having known his guidance through opportunities and a dream, and seen his response to my intimate prayers during my post-viral illness, so I knew I had to keep trusting him even though he was obscured by Despair's darkness and a thick fog of anxiety. I uttered in my soul, 'God, give me the strength to keep on living.'

I thought about the past year and how our trauma and my depression had cut me off from those around me. Shortly after Katherine was born, some of the mothers from our antenatal group had decided to form a social group. I was told that, if I wanted to join, I had to attend the next post-natal coffee morning, as there were too many people to include everyone. The people who attended would form a closed group.

Katherine was still recovering from her operation at the time and we had not developed any kind of set routine. We would leave the house when we were ready, and at a time dictated by the previous night's sleep or lack of it. The appointed morning arrived but, after a terrible night, I struggled to organize myself and after a while conceded that we would not make it on time. I felt angry and hurt. Such a trivial rule was beyond me. The group formed and nobody ever asked me why we did not turn up on the appointed day. I could have asked for a special dispensation, but felt that their lack of understanding was an indicator that we would struggle to meet the group's requirements. I lost a lot of early friendships through this, another cruel consequence of our traumatic beginning.

I decided to attend two local mother-and-toddler groups each week, one at my own church and the other in a hall. However, I found them both difficult. Part of the challenge was that I knew few people with children in our church, so I was completely new to the people there, and in my depression I was not functioning normally. Little things I normally took for granted eluded me. For example, I had always prided myself on being able to get on with anyone, but now in depression I found it much harder. It was as if my 'fall' had changed me, knocking grace and mercy out of me, and all of a sudden I had become an angry, direct and bristly person who was not easy to talk to. I found it hard to discuss things that were important to other mothers but not so vital to me, such as their favourite make of baby clothes or how often their baby slept through the night. These things seemed so trivial compared with my fear for Katherine's survival that I struggled to engage gracefully in conversation, and my inability to do so cut me off from those around me.

The church group was very large, and attracted many women from its affluent neighbourhood. It functioned as an outreach group to the community and provided a communal place for women to meet for coffee, with play equipment and activities for toddlers. Many attended, mainly nannies and local professional mothers, and I felt so small when they described their high-powered jobs or recent skiing trips. I just longed to speak honestly and share my feelings. As time went on, I felt the agreed language of this group was different from mine. Its adjectives were pleasant and superficial, whereas language describing my sad thoughts and deep feelings seemed banned. Although some women there knew that I currently lived in a 'rough place', I felt expected to conform to the dialect of their more comfortable world.

The other group was difficult for the same reason: although desperate to share my pain, I felt required to conceal it. One day I blurted out to a mum I had never met before that Katherine had been very ill and that I was suffering from post-natal depression. The look of horror on her face again reinforced the boundary: attendance at these 'clubs' meant hiding your pain. She never spoke to me again, but just smiled awkwardly from a distance. I longed for someone to really listen and spend time with me so that they would learn the language of my wild place and be able to understand my nuances of desperation.

It was unbearable to be back in an even deeper fog of depression, especially as I had been so close to leaving it behind and realizing my dream of trying for another child. My mind continued to torment me with its most inappropriate and terrifying thoughts. I was deeply shaken by my recent meeting with Despair. Hadn't God promised to protect me from such encounters?

7 'I'm a Christian – get me out of here!'

Deep passionate emotions force us to face questions we would
rather ignore.
Joni Eareckson Tada and Steven Estes[1]

It was as if shockwaves from my encounter with Despair had
shaken the foundations of my faith. I felt the soil beneath
me giving way as I fell deeper and deeper into anger, anxiety
and fear. These deep, passionate emotions were about to
force me to face questions I would rather have ignored.

My fury had started the day Katherine's heart stopped
in hospital. Instantly I felt drawn into a situation I could
not cope with: I had been so profoundly distressed to
witness her death and have to await her resuscitation that
it seemed as if this trauma had caused a violent blow to my
head, which had fractured my mind. My ensuing mental dis-
integration confirmed my belief that this event had been
too much for me. Consequently, I now felt let down by the
Bible where it says, 'No temptation/test[2] has overtaken you
except what is common to us all. God is faithful; he will not
let you be tempted beyond that you can bear, but when you
are tempted he will also provide a way out so that you can

endure it' (1 Corinthians 10:13, TNIV). So I asked God, 'Why was I not provided with "a way out" before I was pushed beyond what I could endure?'

All my life I had clung to that verse as an insurance policy against being overwhelmed. I had thought that if God allowed me to be overcome by a situation, i.e. tempted beyond my limits, I might be forced to take my own life, and that, I knew, would never be his will. So I reckoned that I would experience suffering only in the same measure as I was given strength to endure it. Before these recent challenges, I had piously imagined myself facing barbaric premature death as a missionary and still gracefully submitting to the authority of God, like Jesus in Gethsemane when he said, 'My father, if it is possible, may this cup be taken from me. Yet not as I will, but as you will.'[3] So I was disconcerted (to say the least) to find myself in a much less serious situation and not feeling able to cope.

It was as if I imagined a church at the end of every crisis or precipice, and beyond it a deep, dark pit where Despair and his followers lived, holding people captive. I believed that, as a Christian, all I had to do was run into church where, while meeting with God and his people, I would find protection from being pushed *beyond the edge*. I imagined those who had suffered at the hands of terrorists, for example, as being able to find refuge and strength in God without feeling desperate, and I justified my own escape from childhood horror as a token of being under God's protection. Previously I had envisaged people like myself, mentally ill as I now was, as unfortunate, but still able to see and feel God's presence at the top of the precipice.

Therefore I believed that it was only those without a relationship with God who 'reached the end of themselves', and that this was a result of accumulated sinful behaviours in either their own or other people's lives.

In the wake of meeting Despair, I thought God was

treating me in a very unfair way. I saw myself as a loyal, keen follower who had given her life to God almost from the beginning, when a very young child. Since then, apart from a temporary blip in my teens, I had looked to God for guidance in my life. I had given him my blank canvas – my life's potential – and therefore I felt it was only fair to expect something pretty good in return. I imagined that my canvas was going to look like a sampler tapestry at the end of my life: symmetrical and complete with obvious meaning and purpose. My canvas would look more complete and artistic than those handed over in later life, with half a self-made design to work round!

I presented my angst to God mentally, through a visual picture. I had an image of God working on my tapestry, and only the loose threads being visible to me as he sat in his chair leading and guiding my life. I imagined him crafting, and me sitting opposite waiting for the finished master-piece. I saw myself, getting up and walking round to the front of the canvas, looking at it from his perspective and saying, 'I'm sorry, but I don't like what you are doing here. I gave you a blank canvas that had very little on it; you could have made something beautiful out of it, but now it's full of bleak colours, an unrecognizable mass. If I'd known you were going to make it like this, I would have kept it and designed it myself.'

I had never thought my life was going to turn out this way. I had planned to live fully for God, but in a reward-ing way, not as someone who was held captive by fear for the rest of her life. With incredulity, I stomped about. I told God I was not sure that I wanted him to continue weaving, as I had lost confidence in what he had in store. While I did not actually take my canvas away, I left him in a huff, wondering, 'Does being a Christian not guarantee me a life of perfect guidance and thus one with obvious meaning and purpose?'

Until recently, I felt God *had* honoured the promises I had inherited from my teenage holiday almost twenty years earlier, when I learned that, like Elijah on Mount Carmel,[4] I could trust him to guide and intervene in my life, giving it meaning and fulfilling his purposes. I could see that, until recently, God had led me on a spiritual and personal journey and that my faith had grown. I had matured from a childish faith that had jumped into nursing with eyes closed and hoping for the best, to one with eyes open, willing to accept hardship (ME and a miscarriage) as part of his plan, with faith and grace. I had even felt 'sent' on a variety of occasions: into nursing, to England, back to Northern Ireland and to Colorado, and had been led into marriage and back to England again. Steve and I had both shown a faithful and willing spirit throughout our difficulties.

But now, in my thirty-fourth year, I felt that God was ignoring me. 'Surely', I mused, 'it can't be God's will that I inhabit the wild chaos of anxiety and post-natal depression which renders me unable to be the hopeful, trusting mother and wife I want to be?'

Surely he would not want me to experience such powerful negative emotions, which are the antithesis of my faith. As long as I sought God, confessed my sins and endeavoured to follow his leading, wasn't I guaranteed a life of faith, hope and trust?

And even if I dared to think that God had somehow allowed me to enter into this messy place for some unknown reason, I felt adamant that now was the time to leave. I loved reading about healings in the Bible: how Jesus cured the woman who had been bleeding for twelve years[5] and commended her on her faith in reaching out to him, and how Peter healed Aeneas who had been paralysed for eight years.[6] I had asked many friends all over the world to pray for my healing. Steve and I entreated God constantly as we battled to survive each day. I just loved the idea of God showing his power and glory through a miracle in my life.

For the first time in my life, I felt cut off from God and unable to contact him in my usual ways. Normally, as well as meeting him through Bible reading, prayer and keeping a journal, I could sense God with me, as though his shadow moved ahead of me. Part of this 'sensing', I think, was being aware of his Holy Spirit: feeling led, meeting people at the 'right' time, seeing life events come together with meaning, and recognizing little miracles in ordinary situations. For example, if I was feeling anxious because I had too much to do, often after I had prayed about it others would cancel meetings unexpectedly, leaving me with a sense that God was responding to my requests. However, in my anxiety and depression, I could not sense God in this way.

It was as if I was marooned in a wild and barren place enshrouded in fog and, even though inside I was screaming for help, I could not hear a reply. Indeed, in my worst moments, it was impossible to hear, see or feel anything beyond my captors' presence. The taunts were most audible when I was at home, tired and least distracted, which gave me a critical need to meet God at church. However, this too was difficult, because, as in the other groups, I couldn't find a chance to converse in my new dialect.

Some time ago, Steve and I had decided to give up leading our housegroup because, although we loved the folk in it, we both felt that we could no longer manage to support others spiritually. We discussed it with the members and all agreed to join different groups. Within the new group the people were lovely, so my only problem was that it focused on Bible discussion, with little emphasis on personal matters. I felt as if I was going to burst as I tried to keep my angst to myself. In the end, I found it too difficult to go while being obliged to bury my pain, so I left.

The week before seeing the psychiatrist, when I was feeling particularly low, I had decided to ask God again for some help, so I went along to the church prayer meeting. With tears close, I entered the hall and searched for a friendly face. I could not see anyone I knew well, so I just pulled up a chair, and picked up a leaflet which listed the prayer requests. The evening was all mapped out. I scanned the list to see when I could offer my own requests to God, even wondering whether I would be able to wait until then before asking for help. But I was surprised to discover that there was no opportunity for personal prayer, something I had failed to notice on previous occasions when I had been less needy. Prayer was for those who were not present, not for one another. I felt too upset to pray for the nation or local community projects. What I needed was to ask God if he would somehow help get me through the night.

The intercessions started, and I felt unable to follow what was being said, or pray in the way that others did. People prayed sincerely, but in response to the distant needs of others. Panicked, I got up and left, hoping that someone would see me leave and follow me out. Nobody did. Instead, I sat in the car, howling to God, before starting my short drive home. It seemed that I was not expected to have personal concerns, and nobody else at church had problems or a need to cry out from their heart to God.

The other difficult aspect of my new language was that I seemed to have lost all ability to comprehend or relate to the old one. Before my fall, I loved hearing articulate sermons and eloquently presented theological arguments in our church services, but now I struggled to make sense of them. I loved our church building. It was a beautiful example of a large, formal, sacred space in which to worship God, and it felt so good to enter its familiar walls. I felt safer, and God seemed closer, as soon as I looked at the beautiful stained-glass windows and heard his name being exalted. However, increasingly I was becoming upset. It was as if the service was being conducted in a foreign dialect and I had to strain with my whole being to get the gist of it. I realized that what was being said was very different from my own experience of Christian faith at that time, and I simply could not relate to it.

The sermons were too complex for my fractured mind. They seemed to have been written for those who enjoyed sound mental health, as they did not reflect my mayhem, nor could I act on their instruction. I could not serve others, I could not give more money, I could not encourage Christians, or share my faith with unconverted people, I could not 'do' what I was advised to do in order to keep my faith growing. Nobody referred to the things that were consuming me: anger and disappointment with God's direction in my life, or the jealousy and resentment I felt towards my fellow Christians who were not suffering like my family.

This was also evident in church-family interviews in which people would be brought up to the front. I found my faith wavering in the face of endless reports of personal victories. Although people appeared to be sharing genuine testimonies, they always stated that their misery occurred *before* meeting God, and described their ensuing joy and satisfaction after meeting him. I wondered where I had gone wrong.

It seemed that the rhetoric of my church did not reflect my daily reality, and listening to it increased my sense of alienation from God and from his people. I felt cut off from my faith, my church family and local community groups because there was no natural opportunity to express my new language – my honest desperation – as I struggled to communicate with others the way I had done, by making cheerful, pleasant conversation. In the end, I avoided conversations on a Sunday morning, thus adding to my feelings of isolation, and driving me deeper and deeper into my pit.

Church had become my main community. Now that I was a long way from most of my friends in Ireland who had known me well, I missed having people around who believed in me, and from whom I could receive the support and reassurance I needed. Also, I missed working in a team, and had lost contact with my colleagues at Social Services since being ill and leaving paid employment. This made my need for meaningful relationships at church all the greater. Because the psychiatrists seemed to have little certainty to offer, I believed more than ever that only God could help me get through my anxiety and depression.

'But where can I go to cry out to God and understand his perspective?' I asked. Night after night I thrashed around in the company of torturing accusations from my captors who continued to goad me: I was intrinsically deficient, too unsafe to be an adequate mother, and now too wild to be a child of God. I imagined lying looking upwards at my church on the precipice, and praying for people to don their climbing gear, enter my wild place, and spend time with me far down in my deep crater.

In my mind's eye, I could see the lights of the church in the distance, and shadows of movement in the night sky, as I thought of all the evening meetings that were designed to train others to become spiritually fit: Bible studies, prayer meetings, evangelistic meetings, advanced-discipleship courses, all tailored to prepare them for the day when they would be ready to put on their harnesses and climb down the precipice to rescue a lost soul. There seemed to be so little emphasis on supporting Christians 'in the wild'.

That night, my body ached so much from the wear and tear of my rough terrain that, even if I had not been captive, I would have felt too weak to walk to church. I imagined needing a wheelchair to reach my destination, to support the burden of my brokenness, and visualized arriving at the church steps and ramming my wheels against their concrete, unable to enter the building.

Back in my armchair, I cried with desperation. I looked around my living room on that dark November evening, acknowledging the shadow of Despair, the captors' voices, and the foggy atmosphere of my mind. I looked towards the light, representing a church on the horizon, and cried out to God and his people, 'Please help me. I'm a Christian – get me out of here!' My deep passionate emotions had forced me to face questions I would rather have ignored.

8 Sustenance in the wild

The virtue lies
In the struggle, not the prize . . .
Richard Monckton Milnes (1809–1885)

What I longed for most of all was for my church to be an oasis *as well as* a place of training. I longed for people to be available during the day and in the evening, so that I would have a community I could be with in my desperation. I no longer wanted to share the minutiae of my mind – I had a psychiatrist for that, and felt too vulnerable to have one individual visit me at home, in case they did not understand my terrors. I just longed for regular opportunities to lament to my heavenly Father, without the pressure of outstaying the allotted fifteen minutes. Rather than a GP-appointment slot with God, I wanted a private consultation. I wanted time to uncover my wounds, mourn their pain and lift my arms to God in a plea for help. I needed others to support my weak limbs as 'I presented my requests to God'.[1]

Also, I longed to discuss the gap between my faith and my reality, without judgment or instruction. I wanted to spend time with Christians who would trust God to bring me out of my darkness, yet at the same time I felt afraid that they would not understand that I could not leave it on demand. Although Steve and I often prayed together, I did not want to add to his load, as he was already supporting me in so many ways. He was too close to me, and I wanted independent prayer where I had the freedom to sob without hurting the one who passed the tissues!

Captive again, I feared that I would not be able to maintain my stance against Despair. I desperately wanted to survive, but I also wanted to make the most of my life, for the sake of my gorgeous child. Somehow I realized that success would lie in how I managed my struggle. I prayed for protection from my captors and decided to seek the help I needed.

I opted to take the advice of the doctor and increase my tablets immediately. As I curled up in my living room armchair, my heart sank as I contemplated more months of medication. 'At least this time I have the benefit of hindsight,' I told myself, as I remembered how these tablets had helped me before. Ultimately, I needed to loosen the grip of these thoughts on me, and I felt that my new interrogators had left me with no choice – I had to silence them in whatever way I could.

Steve came in with a glass of milk for me, and we curled up on the sofa together and chatted about the day. We both agreed that I had little option but to increase the dose in the hope that the tablets would make me feel better. Later, I walked into the kitchen, swallowed my three extra capsules and went upstairs to check on Katherine. She looked so beautiful as she slept, that I vowed silently, 'I will overcome this, for your sake and your dad's.' In bed, Steve prayed for God to meet me in my fears and sustain us as a family. My mind still felt on high alert, hyper-stimulated, checking for any signs of evil. I felt so unsure of who I was and what I was capable of, yet, as Steve put his arm around me, I fell asleep, grateful that my husband was not leaving me to cope with these feelings of fear alone.

Steve played a vital role in my support, and I knew I was very fortunate to have a partner who was able to adapt to our circumstances. Instinctively, he seemed to know what kind of help I needed. During a crisis, people often need different things: some may require acts of kindness over and above emotional support; others may desire gifts or physical touch. I believe it depends on one's circumstances and one's 'love language'.[2] However, the most important thing for me was to be listened to and accepted, no matter what.

Despite all our difficulties, Steve chose to stick by me and support me through my fears. He trusted me despite my loss of self-confidence, accepting me at all times rather than becoming my counsellor and trying to work me out (which is probably what I would have done to him!). This made me feel loved and secure in our relationship, and helped strengthen my resolve to overcome my illness for the sake our family.

Steve also helped me in lots of practical ways, particularly during the first few weeks of my relapse, when I was again unable to attend to our household needs due to my constant preoccupation with my anxieties. Often he would arrive home sometime after 6 pm and find me lying on the sofa, with Katherine on the floor surrounded by toys. The television was on as I lay, immobilized by exhaustion and emotional pain. I was unable to follow our normal routine and take Katherine shopping to our local supermarket a hundred yards away. So Katherine and I waited for Steve to return, tired and worn out. He would always enter the room cheerfully and exude joy on seeing his precious daughter. Only then would I feel guilty that I had not found the energy to sort things out for dinner, but had lain helplessly, waiting for his return. Often I did not notice the chaos of the room until I saw it through his eyes, as he surveyed the devastation. Graciously, he would ask if we needed some food. As he shut the door behind him, I would look at Katherine with tears in my eyes, wondering why I felt unable to be the capable mother and wife I so wanted to be.

The timing of my relapse made things even more difficult for me. Katherine was older now and had more energy, and I was weary from losing my fight with my terrors. When I had first become depressed, Katherine was only six months old, and during the day she was quite easy to look after. She played happily in her baby gym and was easily amused in cafés and shops. She took regular naps, which gave me the opportunity to catch up on lost sleep or just rest. But now, a year later, she was an active toddler and, in my relapsed state, I found her hard to care for. Often I was irritable with my gorgeous child and found her incessant need for activity annoying. I just wanted to go to sleep and find release from my mental torture, but instead I had to try to entertain her. Sadly, during those weeks we did not play a lot, but watched too much poor-quality TV.

However, even in my weak condition, I did try to help Steve, to compensate for his hard work. I ensured that he slept well and took regular breaks, so that he could maintain his health. It was one thing for me to have crashed as a person, but I recognized that, if Steve fell apart too, our family life would crumble. Consequently, I always nursed Katherine through her night-time pain and tried to ensure that he got some time to himself at weekends to recharge his batteries. As an aeronautical engineer, he travelled all around the world and, although I worked part-time, Katherine and I were financially dependent on his salary.

During my relapse, I found it difficult when Steve had to travel to France for a couple of days. One Monday morning, at five o'clock, I sat crying on the stairs as he ran round the house trying to pack. When he came down, I told him that

I did not think I could manage without him, and that I felt afraid of being left alone with Katherine. Steve turned round and, looking at me lovingly, told me that he was sorry but he had to go, and that he believed I would be able to manage without him. As he closed the door, I wept in the darkness of the winter morning as I turned to go back to bed. I resented his ability to leave my fears behind, and my *lack of* ability to escape from them! My depression was now like a sick game of hide and seek in which, having been pushed into rough terrain, I was now expected to find the cleverly concealed escape route through some cunning plan of my own. I was getting tired of playing, as the exit was continually out of my reach, and yet Steve and the others who came to visit me seemed able to come and go quite casually.

Steve's steadiness was like a rock onto which I could hold: a steadiness not just in himself but also in his faith in God. He had already passed through his own dark time of questioning when his mother had died so young and, after finding his answers his faith, had been restored. Now he was able to understand and accept my spiritual thrashing around, so he displayed a quiet confidence that God would be faithful to us in our suffering. Sometimes I was very hard to live with, yet he showed me mercy and grace, with the reassurance that we would survive the battering.

Despite loving my parents very much, I found it very difficult to talk to them about my depressive feelings on the telephone: I did not want to worry them when they were in their seventh decade of life and living so far away. So when they rang to ask how I was managing without Steve, I explained briefly that I was feeling anxious again and that I needed to go back on a higher dose of my tablets. They responded with concern and offered to visit, but I explained that I did not feel up to visitors, as I was barely able to manage my own external world for Katherine and myself.

Sensing my struggle, Mum persisted with her enquiries: 'What way does this make you feel, and how does it affect you?'

'I feel totally exhausted,' I explained. 'The increased dose really knocks me out, and Katherine is not sleeping very well.' I omitted to mention that my body was also worn out from tension as I constantly relived worst-case scenarios in my head while waiting for my medication to work. 'Your dad and I are praying for you, and I have asked other friends, some of whom have a special healing ministry, to pray for you too.' Sympathetically, Mum went on to ask me how was I coping with practical chores such as cooking, cleaning and ironing. I explained that I was really struggling. Two days later I received a lovely note from her and a cheque from Dad. 'Please use this money to get some help with the house while you are feeling so ill,' the note said.

My father-in-law was also very supportive. He rang us regularly and kept in close contact. He too understood the impact of my illness on our family life, and willingly contributed to our finances. Our parents' financial gifts were an amazing blessing to us, enabling us to buy ready-made meals when we were both too weary to cook, and to employ a regular cleaner. Although physically absent, our parents made their support tangible to us. Many others were supportive too. I had regular phone-calls from my brothers and sisters-in-law, and other friends both locally and in Ireland.

Within a few weeks, I noticed a gradual improvement, a loosening of the grip of my fears. Now I was able to change Katherine's nappy without feeling such constant terror and, although my acute self-doubt persisted, I felt less threatened by it. It was as if I had been given a foothold out of my crater and was now walking on uneven ground. I was now able to think about things other than my obsessional fears.

So taking a therapeutic dose of Prothiaden again *did* give me some respite from my mental torture, as if my captors had given me a tagging device. It did not give me total freedom from my feral place, but it did give me increased movement and mobility within a wider perimeter. I felt as if I was being released from my crater during the day, but returning to it at night, when my accusers would cross-examine me for proof of my innocence.

Soon I realized that, although the tablets were reducing the immense feeling of threat, unfortunately this time they did not take my scary thoughts away. Rather, I would not allow myself to believe that the presence of these thoughts was due solely to my depression. My need to work them out was at odds with the taking of this particular medication, as it slowed down my mental processes and I was unable to force myself to regain mental clarity. Although I found it unbearable to lose lucidity, this course of treatment was partially effective for me and I believe I would have survived less well without it. Despair stood close during the evenings and I had to hold firmly to my knowledge of God in order to resist his offering of oblivion.

'Try reading Dorothy Rowe's book,' said a close friend. 'I have heard it gives an accurate account of depression. I was frantic for information, as I needed to understand what was happening to me. Reading *Depression – The Way Out of Your Prison*[3] was such a comfort to me. Finally I knew that somebody else understood how I felt, and immediately it seemed less scary. This book gave an accurate account of the horror of my captivity and offered me an explanation of how I had arrived there and how I could escape. Rowe described depression as a prison and suggested that its walls are built throughout one's life, but that depression finally arrives in its fullness when something comes along and closes the door. There was no doubt in my mind that Katherine's cardiac arrest had secured my entrance into captivity, but I was unsure how the walls had been built. I found one phrase particularly helpful: 'Not trusting yourself has rendered you helpless'.[4] Somehow I had to stop looking to others for reassurance and begin to trust myself again. I felt thankful to God for using the discipline of psychology, through Rowe's book, to shed some light and help me take a few more steps towards the exit.

During this time, I was still attending Psychiatric Outpatients. My young doctor, whom I saw a couple of times, left for a new post elsewhere and I was assigned to another young physician. Pleasant in manner, he frustrated me with his preoccupation with the practical details of my life – how much sleep I was getting at night, and how many times my husband attended to Katherine's nightly needs – rather than helping me deal with my frightening anxieties. I felt he was missing the point so, at my request, I was assigned to the care of another, more experienced, doctor.

But I was soon to discover that experience is not always a guarantee of a satisfying relationship. Arriving late, this middle-aged female doctor made no apology, and then greeted me with a very measured smile. She managed our introductions in a formal, cold and non-empathetic manner and I wondered how on earth I was going to entrust this person with my most intimate and terrifying thoughts. Although I had now been on a full dose of medication for three months, I was still being tortured nightly during my curfew, and desperately needed to share my disturbing thoughts with her.

Reluctantly, I did eventually describe them to her, as my need to talk about my fears exceeded my need to be accepted by her. She listened attentively, without flinching, as I shared my arduous journey, and responded by looking blankly back at me. I was not comforted by this encounter and did not know what it meant. When I ended my soliloquy, this doctor merely nodded, and the only comfort I gained from her was that she planned to see me again in two months' time, without suggesting that she would ring Social Services in the meantime. Her lack of feedback and analysis made me wonder, 'What is the purpose of this visit? Does this doctor envisage her role merely as that of a sounding board or a screening system to check my likelihood of self-harm or danger to others?'

Yet, strangely, she did eventually provide me with some companionship as she became familiar with my feral place. She offered me bi-monthly appointments, which gave me the opportunity to be more honest than I could be in most other relationships. Here I did not have to pretend that my daily habitat was light and easy; she knew my toil, was familiar with my fears, and, most importantly, was not frightened by them. Although I did not receive emotional warmth from her, I felt believed and trusted by her. Curiously, I discovered that her attitude to me and my terrors helped me to endure them, as on hearing of them she was not instructing me to pack my bag and leave the family home.

The only other place where I could be fairly honest was in a group organized by church members that met in a home. It was a mums' group that met once a week for Bible study and prayer, while kind volunteers looked after our children in another room. When I joined initially, as at the previously mentioned church groups I felt quite out of it. The other women seemed so 'sorted' and I felt such a wreck. However, once I had the courage to say I was suffering from post-natal depression, I discovered that two out of the other ten were also suffering from it! The form the depression took was quite different in each case and, although I did not share the details of my fears with this group, I did at least feel totally accepted in my brokenness.

Over time I became soulmates with some of these women, and learned that they, like me, felt marooned in a wild place. Together we laughed, cried and prayed as we supported one another through depression, serious childhood illnesses and relationship difficulties, and often around feeding babies, and in spite of limited quality time. Our leaders were sensitive to our varying needs and tried their best to share simple biblical truths creatively, and leave enough time for personal support. The Bible study itself was important to me, as I found it easier to understand by talking it through. In the group we were helped by the knowledge that we were not the only ones who were cut off. However, because of our own needs and struggles, most of us were unable to support one another as we wanted to. So, while I really appreciated and valued the support I gained from this group, it was not enough to sustain me throughout the week. Also, because of the nature of my particular anxieties, I did not feel I could share them there.

Having friends at church who knew something of my struggles and could converse with me on a deeper level really helped me to attend, even though I felt on the margins. I now felt less alone and more able to gain something positive from the services, and seeing many others in corporate worship strengthened my resolve to reject Despair. Gradually, as I grew stronger, I found that if I made a commitment to attend each week, I did gain some sustenance: through a line from a song, a prayer, a Bible reading, a talk or a conversation.

While my prayer life consisted mostly of frequent, short, pleading prayers, or conversations in my head while walking Katherine in the pram, it was nonetheless vital to me. I prayed regular desperate prayers for protection from Despair: that he would not overcome me and that God would enable me to maintain my stance against him until I could see the way out. Also, I chatted frankly to God, and on more than one occasion told him that he had better have something great planned as a result of my awful depression! Although I did not know what God was doing, I still believed that he was doing something useful and that it was within his power to protect me and lead me onto a better path.

Soon we had additional challenges: Katherine's nightly abdominal pain seemed to be getting worse. We saw her consultant and described what our nights were like: Katherine would wake up regularly, and would writhe and roll about the bed, arching her back and screaming at high volume. When Steve or I tried to comfort her, she would kick and push us off the bed, and we would end up pacing the house, arguing over what to do next. She did not seem to be awake at these times and yet seemed in genuine pain. We both found these episodes very distressing.

I found it very hard to rouse myself in the first place, as if I was calling myself back from a deep, heavy-sedated sleep. As I dragged myself over the metre of carpet between Katherine and me, I felt as if I was being ripped apart as I watched my precious daughter grow hysterical. We tried the softly, softly approach: 'There, there, Mum and Dad are with you', but also resorted to 'What is wrong with you? Why don't you just stop crying?' Some nights I feared for the neighbours' sanity, and I struggled to carry Katherine downstairs to muffle her screams as she clung to the banisters. Sympathetic and concerned, the consultant ordered an investigation into her reflux and said it would be carried out in a few weeks' time.

Following a test whereby she had a tube inserted up her nose and into her stomach for twenty-four hours, it was discovered that Katherine was refluxing acid, rather than an alkaline fluid which was more common. This shed some light on her night-time crying. She was given new medication and a few weeks later we were amazed to see how well she could sleep! Her wakefulness did not disappear completely, however, but improved greatly with this medication.

The following months were difficult as I came to terms with my chronic condition and tried to accept that Katherine was growing up in my wild place. I was a perfectionist and, as far as I was concerned, it was just not good enough that her formative years were being spent with someone in captivity. The whole situation was intolerable, but I had no choice. I could not get out of my depression, and I could not bear to leave Katherine with a childminder or in a nursery, and I was not fit to go to back to work as a social worker. I had to wait until I was able to find my own exit before I could bring about her release. I had to make the best of the struggle, actively fighting it, as I believed that we would survive it less well if I passively gave in.

At least my medication gave me more opportunities to take Katherine into brighter places, even though I could still hear the murmurings of my captors' voices. Also, I discovered that doing regular activities each day helped me to achieve things despite my mood. So we attended the toddler groups that Katherine enjoyed. Thankfully, she loved going to work with me, as she had a friend and lots of great toys to play with, so our mornings were easily catered for. Afternoons posed more challenges, as my energy tended to wane. I tried to get to the supermarket when I needed to, and meet friends as often as possible, and we occasionally looked after one another's children, though unfortunately this was difficult as I was finding it hard to take risks, even for my closest friends.

One of the more positive results of my depression was learning that the discipline of doing things despite feeling terrible was beneficial. I learned to embrace life even though it was not perfect. Steve, Katherine and I had some really good times together, and also with family and friends, while I was in my wild place, for I learned that as long as I was courageous enough to leave my crater, i.e. my home, my captors did not have total control over me.

I found it was important to try to have balance in my day, to get out and do something enjoyable for Katherine's sake, and to rest if possible. If Katherine would not sleep I would let her play in her cot for an hour, while I lay on my bed.

Being honest about our respective needs was refreshing and helped me to find energy to endure the struggle.

There were times when Steve was at work and I could not manage on my own and needed the practical help of others. I believe that God provided for me at such times through the availability of the hands and voices of others. However, this often required that I swallow my pride and ring a family member or a friend to ask for support in the form of a vital chat on the phone or a visit. I found it very hard to ask but, when I did, I felt as if those who responded were 'angels unaware'.

Help came like manna:[5] on a daily basis, rather than in stockpiles in advance. Often I had to go out and fetch it, or make decisions to do things I did not feel like doing. On those days I felt as if I was on my knees clawing sustenance from a parched land. Yet, at other times, family and friends freely gave us what we needed, as if handing it to us on a plate!

The foggy, dark, captive days of my depression seemed endless. It would have been unfair though to my precious child and loving husband if I had given up the struggle to be my best before the prize of my release. Contrary to my fears and, though I was unable to see it at the time, I did find enough help to maintain my stance against Despair. I found the strength to endure my rough terrain in the belief that there was a way out and a better road awaited me.

9 Risking escape

Courage is only an accumulation of small steps.
George Konrad (1993)[1]

Eight months after my relapse, I became desperate to hatch another escape plan, though my cerebral captors roared with laughter at the very notion: 'Go on, try it; let's see how far you get this time, but when you fail we are really going to let you have it!' I felt terrified at the thought of another foiled attempt, as my last fall had hurt *so* much: my relapse had taken me to an even more scary place than before and I wondered, 'Could things get any worse if I failed again?'

It was as if the recent months of moving around my rough terrain had led me to a new rock face. I had taken enough small steps out of my crater, out of the total control of my anxieties, to give me the courage to take even more steps towards change.

I was fortunate to have a strong motivating factor: my desire for another child, a sibling for Katherine, which drove me like a powerful engine. Without that burning desire, I might never again have ventured off solid ground or taken risks in my bid for freedom, but I had no choice. My maternal heartstrings constantly reverberated within me and I could no longer bear the din. I had to proceed towards pregnancy, which as far as I was concerned meant trying to come off medication. But I did not want to embark on another pregnancy without having recovered from my last bout of depression. I needed to know that I could recover and leave my wild place.

I felt I was being reasonable, not rash. I discussed it with my psychiatrist, who nodded wisely, 'Yes, fine, if you think you are up to it.'

'Why is it always down to me?' I complained to Steve. 'No-one seems to be able to tell me what to do. I always have to try and figure it out for myself and find out when I am ready, and I don't know! Look what happened last time!' We both felt lost, as nobody seemed to be able to offer any clear direction. Everything was so woolly, so full of mights or maybes.

My new honest self started to talk: 'It is going to be difficult, as you are on six tablets a day and you have become dependent on them for managing your anxious thoughts. You will need to make life as easy as possible so that you can endure the harshness of your climate. Think about what you can do to help yourself.'

'I need to give up work,' I said to Steve. 'I think I need a break to help me recover from my depression, particularly now that I am going to come off medication – I need to slow down.' The last two years had taken their toll and I was feeling shattered most of the time. Although Katherine's sleeping had improved, she still woke up very distressed during the night at least three to four times a week and that, combined with the constant activity at work, was making me really tired.

Steve and I discussed things long into the night, and agreed that maybe it was time for Katherine to start nursery part-time. I could use that time to rest. We could remortgage our house to release some capital, at least to pay for nursery fees and the loss of income in the short term.

We set things in motion, and I gave in my notice at work with very mixed feelings. James had become my friend as well as my employer, and I knew that Katherine and I would miss our regular contact with him and his family, but I felt the time was right. I needed to change my routine, and felt that it would be good for Katherine to learn to be independent from me and socialize more with other children.

The weeks went by quickly, and soon I had finished work and only the summer lay between Katherine and nursery. We enjoyed a family holiday in Scotland and then Katherine and I had one week in Jersey with my parents, where another problem developed right out of the blue: Katherine developed severe eczema. The sea water and sand irritated her fair skin and, despite her love for the beach, we had to avoid it. Her ankles were red and raw, and her whole body covered in a prickly rash. Towards the middle of the week, she developed a nasty infection in her wrist and was prescribed antibiotics by a local doctor. I sat on the floor crying as Katherine flung the syringe full of medicine across the room. 'Lord,' I prayed, 'why is life so hard?'

Back home, we struggled to control Katherine's skin infection as she prepared to go to nursery, but our local GP became concerned at its persistence and referred her to a dermatologist.

Now, as the time approached for Katherine to go to nursery, I was feeling more and more empty. Over the past two and a half years, my life had been so consumed by her survival that I could not bear the thought of being without her. The day duly arrived, and I felt as if someone was removing my heart. Leaving each other was traumatic for both of us. Katherine cried as I left, and I felt gripped with a terror that I would never see her again. I felt my accusers homing in on me and reminding me of our precarious life to date: 'Bad things happen to you – are you sure you can really trust these people to look after your only child?'

During the past four years I had felt as if I was wearing a magnetic device that attracted trouble. I was afraid of trying out new things in case I encouraged even more. Now, with the knowledge that God allows his children to fall and be held captive by despair, I felt afraid of life in case he brought me back to that unbearable place. Hypervigilance took over as I screened life for trouble. Never again did I want to be floored by another bombshell!

Until this moment, I had not realized just how much *I* needed to be with Katherine, to reassure myself of her survival, so letting go, even for a few hours, was excruciating. Life seemed so dull without her, as I walked round my neighbourhood feeling empty. Then I started noticing others around me, and it seemed as if every woman in the street was either pregnant or pushing a newborn baby in a pram. 'I can't stand this; I need to do something with my free time or I will go crazy!' I said.

Yet nothing interested me. All I wanted was to have another baby and provide Katherine with the sibling she deserved. How could I attend to anything else when it all seemed so trivial? But I knew I would have to try to find something that would give me purpose, as the emptiness I felt was unbearable. All my friends either had other children or jobs, and I knew I would not climb out of my depression if I stayed in this empty place.

'Social work? No way!' I thought. 'I can barely cope with my *own* problems, never mind anyone else's. Retail? No, I still don't feel well enough to get myself up and out to work. A course?' I continued quizzing myself. 'Maybe, but I feel so depressed, I don't think anything could hold my attention and motivate me to go.' I felt leaden with grief, as if wearing protective X-ray clothing. I so much wanted to move on, but I just couldn't. 'Sign language, Deaf Studies?' Now a glimmer of light was appearing. I did have a genuine interest in Deaf people and their fascinating language, so could this woo me into life again?

I started to research the possibilities and discovered there was a part-time Master's course in Deaf Studies at the university one mile from my home, and half a mile from Katherine's nursery. 'Perfect.' I so wanted to stop taking my medication but was scared of doing this. Perhaps the distraction and the challenge would help me to take the risk? I immediately applied for the course and was accepted. Katherine was now settling into nursery, and I was coping better with my free time, knowing that soon I was going to be doing something interesting.

Two weeks before my course started, I reduced my medication by one tablet. So far so good: I had taken my first step onto the rock face. I did not notice a vast difference and hoped that coming off medication second time round was going to be swift and smooth.

I arrived at the Deaf Studies Department a fortnight later, feeling optimistic as I took more risks and moved further up my crag. However, I was unprepared for the challenge that lay ahead. With very little memory of my stage-one British sign-language vocabulary, I felt overwhelmed when I entered the signing environment. 'Voices off,' we were told, and I floundered as I dragged the remnants of my basic sign-language skills to the forefront of my mind. 'Is this how Deaf people feel in the hearing world?' I wondered, panicked and confused by my inability to communicate with anyone. Over fifty students had gathered for the induction lecture and, in spite of the fixed grin on my face, I felt internal terror return with a vengeance.

My mind struggled to cope with the constant stimulation, and my remaining 125mg dose of Prothiaden did not lend itself to swift cognition. 'The only other thing I want to do apart from have another baby is out of my reach,' I realized, and I felt the presence of Despair tower over me again, as if he was following in hot pursuit.

However, I stayed for the morning session, and ended up whispering my name to the proficient hearing signer I was sitting next to, as he struggled to understand my fumbling hand shapes.

The following week I returned for lectures. As I walked the short distance from Katherine's nursery, I felt torn with conflicting emotions. On the one hand, I was proud to be re-entering academic life and excited about the course, yet on the other, a voice in my heart goaded me regarding the futility of my journey: 'All you want is another baby – what on earth are you doing this for?'

The next two months were challenging as I drove myself to attend lectures despite an overpowering desire to go home and cry because I was not pregnant. My unit was called 'Deaf Studies in Perspective', and as I watched the lecture in BSL and listened to the interpreter's voice, I learned how many signing Deaf people see themselves as a linguistic minority rather than a group of people disabled by hearing loss (as the hearing world tends to define them). I studied Deaf history and learned how so much of their past has been controlled by hearing people, and how they have been disempowered, within education, family life and the church!

Two months later, I reduced my medication by another tablet, to 100mg. I was struggling with concentration and mental agility, and hoped that the fog would lift with another decrease. 'Am I going to be able to write my 3,000-word assignment? Is the medication going to permit these cognitive processes?' I wondered.

It was not long before I had to consider these questions seriously as I struggled with the very real demands of the course. Although I was required to attend only one three-hour lecture a week, most of my fellow students were single and studying full-time. They had good sign-language skills, and I found myself feeling very isolated by my poor signing, time restraints and home responsibilities. In addition, I was using the only two free mornings I had for university or the library, and so had no time to carry out daily chores. I began to recognize that maybe I had bitten off more than I could chew. As I worked all weekend towards my assignment deadline, I resented the enforced separation from Steve and Katherine, and wondered, 'Is this course right for me?'

My answer came at three in the morning a few days later, as Katherine woke up, unsettled and in pain. I needed to finish my assignment later that day and had gone to bed only two hours earlier. Katherine failed to be comforted and, feeling exhausted and frustrated, I picked up her beaker of water and flung it, away from her, across the bedroom, angry that she was keeping me awake on such a crucial night. It bounced and hit the floor, smashing to bits. Katherine immediately stopped crying with the shock of the bang and incredulity at her mother's outburst. I was appalled at how I had frightened her. I rushed over and hugged her, vowing never to throw her cup again. There and then I told myself, 'I will withdraw from the course tomorrow, if I am going to behave like this. It is obviously too much pressure for me.

I was discovering my limits the hard way. Although I was reducing my medication and successfully climbing away from my captors, I felt as though I had underestimated my weakness and tried to move too far, too quickly. I had put my family life and myself at risk, and needed to stop and rethink my strategy. I held on to my reduced dose, but could not go any further. I needed to figure out my pace first.

I managed to complete my assignment and leave the course, having done one unit. Immediately afterwards, in January 2000, I decided to join a British sign language level-two night class, which would develop the production and reception of my sign-language skills. I loved my weekly evenings with our class and my Deaf BSL teacher. It was such good fun and yet required every moment of my fractured mind's attention, forcing me to leave my disturbing thoughts behind. I benefited hugely from the respite, and felt during these classes that I was scrambling higher towards my peak.

As my confidence in my ability to sign at a basic level grew, I decided to sit next to the Deaf people who attended the evening service at our church. Initially I just watched them, but eventually I started to sign to them. I sat with them and signed the worship songs, copying the interpreter. I signed 'God', pointing upwards with my right index finger, and then bringing it directly in front of my upper body and joining my left index finger in the same hand shape to sign 'God with me'. The hairs on my body stood on end as I 'saw' God for the first time in a long time.

It was as if I had just climbed up my rock face, beyond the oppressive mist and fog of my depression, for the very first time. I had recovered enough to allow a reduction in my sedative medication without my symptoms returning, and gained from my small steps into new situations the ability to think and feel again. Once I had arrived at that place, I saw that God *was* beside me after all, only this time he communicated with me in my new language. My eyes glistened with tears at the realization.

Feeling that God was meeting me through this visual language confirmed my belief that he had been with me every step of the way. He already knew that I had a new dialect and was struggling to comprehend the old one. He knew that I needed to see things visually, as my mind was still not functioning normally. I felt accepted, known and loved. No longer did I imagine that God was standing within the church at the top of the precipice, asking, 'How did you get yourself down there? I will not speak to you until you manage to pull yourself up this cliff edge to me.' No, I felt as if God was saying to me, 'Hazel, I never left you. I know you have had a terrible time, been badly injured, struggled to survive, and been able to converse with only a few, but I never left your side. I've been tending your wounds and guiding your steps towards the exit. Often people cannot see or hear me when they go *beyond the edge*.' I felt the warmth of God's presence again, for the first time in a very long while, and my immediate need for answers waned.

Over the next weeks and months, I realized that God had not only given me a new way of relating to him, but also some new companions to relate to. As a result of learning this language, I was developing meaningful relationships with the Deaf members of my church, and we had more in common than I realized. Although they were young, single and enjoying good mental health, within the church we were very similar: unable to take part fully in church life because of the language barrier. They too could not attend the prayer meeting or weekly housegroups, as there was no interpreter available mid-week. Prayer ministry was also difficult for them, as they could only access it when an interpreter was available, and then they were limited to discussing prayer requests they felt comfortable with in the presence of their interpreter. As the notices were being read out and the Deaf members ignored the interpreter and signed to one another, I realized how irrelevant most of the notices were to them. Here were others too who were restricted from full membership of the church. As I worshipped God clumsily with my hands, I marvelled at how he had brought us together and, from that evening on, we started our own Bible study group, using BSL as our first language.

Again I reduced my medication, and my excitement quickened as I considered stopping altogether and trying for another pregnancy. I loved Katherine *so* much and the thought of having another little person like her excited me beyond belief. Yet I was still struggling to be the parent I wanted to be. With every decrease in medication, I experienced increased anxiety, and feared my captors would pull me down by the tag they had attached to me, which as yet I could not remove.

Early in spring, six months after her referral, Katherine received an appointment to see a consultant dermatologist. 'That's good,' I said to Steve, 'as I've noticed her eczema is getting worse again.' It had grumbled on through the winter months, never fully going away. Katherine was again more wakeful at night and I did not know why. Sometimes she writhed, as if in pain, and at other times she just seemed unsettled.

On arrival at the hospital, I did my usual 'pushy-parent' routine and asked if we could see the consultant, much to the embarrassment of my gentle husband. 'There is *only* a consultant in clinic today' I was told, and I breathed a sigh of relief.

'You will need to start bandaging Katherine from head to toe in order to treat and manage her eczema.' I listened in disbelief as the consultant told us that she had widespread eczema that was very itchy, and that, without careful management, it would cause skin damage and she would suffer from recurrent infections. He sent us off with the nurse, who showed us the bandages and explained our new routine. 'Every night you will need to bath Katherine, apply steroid cream to the worst areas and then bandage her with Viscopaste® bandages. They are impregnated with a special cream, and the moisture and heat will help the absorption of the steroid cream. Then you need to cover the bandage with Tubigrip®, which you have to measure in advance, cutting holes for her arms in the body ones.'

'So I have to bandage her whole body as well?'

'Yes. If you look at her body, although it's not bleeding like her arms and legs, it is covered all over in eczema, which is incredibly itchy and will worsen unless treated.'

'How much does God think we can take here?' I retorted to myself. 'In the midst of my coming off antidepressants, we are now expected to wrap our precious child in bandages every night! How on earth will we manage to get a three-year-old to co-operate, and what on earth will it be like for her?'

So a new routine was born, which initially took an hour and a half every evening: placing a wet sheet down, then a chair on top, putting on a video and then wrapping her up. Initially, Katherine was understandably quite freaked out, and both she and I wept as we tried to negotiate our way through the lengthy process. It required co-operation from all three of us: Steve and I drew Katherine's attention to the video as we covered our dear child in swaddling clothes. Amazingly, she adapted quickly, and we discovered that it did in fact help her to sleep, as she seemed more comfortable. I took the bandages off every morning, as they were quite restricting, and we soon got used to having bits of them all over the floor.

Despite this setback, I could see that I was getting close to the top of my cliff. I reduced my medication to two tablets a day and enjoyed an even clearer mind and the ability to look at my situation more rationally. This encouraged my progress and, by the end of September 2000, I had successfully stopped all medication. I was immediately discharged by the psychiatrist and encouraged to follow my dreams. 'I want to get pregnant immediately, Steve. Katherine is three and I really want her to have a sibling as soon as possible, so that it is easy for her to adapt to the change.'

I felt as though I was standing on level ground, but had reached the top. However, it was only now that I could see the other peak in front. Success in climbing this would give me another baby, and I said to myself, 'I have no choice but to step out in faith. I have to negotiate this final rock face to realize my dreams. Lord, here goes! Help me to scale this.'

It was so good to have moved on, to have found the courage through a succession of small steps to climb the rock face out of depression, by reducing my medication and taking limited risks. My new confidence that God was with me, and that he had not left me in recent years, but had just been hidden from view, gave me my first step towards my new peak.

10 Stumbling with excess baggage

Facing fears means facing facts.
Grace Sheppard[1]

'I'm pregnant, Steve.' I showed him the faint blue line. 'My period was due a few days ago, and I thought I would check, just in case.' We both beamed with delight at the thought of another baby. 'I've done it. With your help, I've dared to step towards pregnancy again, and you have seen to the rest. Thank you, God.'

'But I'm not depressed any more, so why am I feeling *so awful*?' I asked Steve. I thought of my friend's words of caution: 'Are you sure you are ready for another pregnancy? You have just stopped your medication and come through a difficult time.' Yet I knew that if I did not jump immediately I would never leap again. If I had stopped to ponder, I would have run in the opposite direction. 'I want another baby for everyone's sake, no matter what,' I told myself.

But now, in the quietness of the early morning, I was struggling with some overpowering thoughts. 'What on earth have you done? You have just crawled out of the captivity of your depression and got off those horrendous drugs, and now you are going to climb another sheer face, and you expect me to be chilled about it?' It was as if I was having an argument with myself and I was completely split in two. Half of me was so relieved that I had taken the risk, but the other half was completely freaked out.

The internal clamour was unbearable, and very quickly my elation was overcome by a dread that I had never known before. I rang some friends and asked them to pray for me, and walked around the house pleading for God to help. While I knew that Steve was concerned for me, I was also delighted to see the lightness in his step and was glad for his sake that I had taken the risk, even if it was killing me.

As the days went on, time seemed to stand still. We didn't tell Katherine, as I was only six weeks pregnant and we feared disappointing her. Yet inside I was floundering, and feeling that I was again slipping down my cliff. 'I'm not ready for this,' was my overwhelming feeling. 'It's as if I am trying to climb with a broken limb and it is not holding up under the pressure. I haven't really sorted out the answers to my fears and here I am getting pregnant all over again. Can I really trust myself? What if my old fears come back to haunt me? What if I have to go back on those awful drugs? *God, please help me.*'

I felt as if my head was going to break, that something within was saying, 'I can't take the mental strain; I am going to snap.' Restful sleep eluded me. I would manage to sleep for a couple of hours, before getting up to rock and pace about with anxiety. I bought a relaxation video and found that, by carrying out its exercises at 2 am, I could sleep for a few more hours.

According to my GP, it was too early for a scan, and I did not confess to him how desperate I was feeling. I came home from my appointment. Katherine was at nursery, so I dialled the number. 'Hello, pregnancy advice line.' I started to cry and pour out my woes to this complete stranger. 'You could come in and talk to one of our advisors about whether you want to carry on with this pregnancy or have an abortion.'

'No I can't,' I snapped back. 'I don't want an abortion. I want this baby, but I just feel overwhelmed and gripped by the fear of what might be ahead of me again.' I put the phone down after our short conversation and wondered what on earth I was going to do. It was good to know that I could talk to people like this, but they did not seem to understand that I could not have an abortion even if I felt overwhelmed. I did not believe God would ever want that of me. Yet I felt as though this pregnancy was pushing me over the edge again, and feared I would lunge back into captivity. Inwardly I was hysterical. Yes, I wanted another child desperately, but not if it meant returning to my wild place. I could not bear to be lost there for another three years. I struggled through the next few days, grumpy and irritable.

However, I started digging deep into my soul for answers and, while walking down to the nursery one day, I had a 'eureka moment'. I realized that part of my problem was that I was carrying excess baggage, and I needed to go back and look at my depressive anxieties and face their core questions. I imagined myself climbing, with a backpack full of parcels. I knew roughly what was inside them: I had taken a brief peek at their size, but had not opened them individually or looked at their contents properly. These parcels were now jumping up and down, calling out for attention and upsetting my balance. Suddenly I realized that I needed to open them and examine what was inside each one, and then I would be less likely to fall backwards off the cliff.

Steve came home that night and I told him of my revelation. 'I think I understand why I am feeling so awful about this pregnancy. I have not faced my fears fully, and have therefore given them the power to keep freaking me out. Even though I still feel scared, I also feel hugely relieved, as I now know what I need to do to cope with this pregnancy.'

The next morning I woke to discover that I was bleeding heavily, and I knew in my heart that it was all over. It was as if I was having an unusually heavy period, and I realized that I was losing the pregnancy. I rang the local maternity unit and they called me in immediately. Katherine went to play with a friend, and Steve and I went to the hospital.

'I am sorry, Mrs Rolston, there is no sign of a pregnancy. I am afraid you have had an early miscarriage, but I am sure you can always try again!' I felt the thump of my landing back on the ledge again.

During the next few days, I felt a whole mixture of emotions: relief that I did not have to deal with the fear of another pregnancy and face the possibility of post-natal depression again, but devastation that my best attempt to rise above life's hurts had failed again. I felt in some ways that God had shown me that he knew my limits, but why had he not given me a foothold and the supernatural strength I needed?

Katherine was now attending playgroup as well as nursery, and I had more time to myself. I was feeling rotten: worn out and beaten up by life. Mixing with Katherine and her friends invariably meant being around other women who were pregnant and had multiple children, and I found it *so* painful. Their ability to carry on a pregnancy was a constant reminder of my loss. The boxes from Charing Cross Oncology Department started to arrive again, as I was checked for the return of a hydatidiform mole. Thankfully, within a couple of months, I was given the all-clear.

One of the hardest things for me at this stage was facing my feelings, as well as rising above them for Katherine's sake. I coped with this by distracting myself and trying to meet Katherine's needs as much as I could, for example by arranging play dates and trips out with friends. However, increasingly, I was feeling very low and I feared that my depression was returning.

'Please could we have regular healing services at our church?' I asked the minister. 'I am really struggling and need some quality time in prayer so that I can really cry out to God for his help.' We talked, and I confessed to him just how hard I had found being a Christian in his church while I was depressed, and how inaccessible many things had seemed to me. I described my brokenness and how I had felt that others did not know how to cope with it. I told him that I felt too abrasively honest for most groups, and had few opportunities to come and offer my lament to God without worrying about whom else I was upsetting. 'Please could we have a separate service, where people can come and just cry in the presence of God? Just be our broken selves and really spend some time pleading for God's intervention?'

I told him of the confusion I felt when I listened to countless 'successful' testimonies, and explained how I needed to know that other people in God's kingdom struggled and suffered too. It all came out that day in a flurry of desperate pleas. 'And, as for sermons,' I went on, 'please think of people who suffer when you preach.'

'Leave it with me,' he said graciously. 'I will get back to you.' I left feeling I had been listened to, but unsure how much would change. However, I received the minister's generous response within a few weeks: 'We are going to have a healing service on Ash Wednesday at 7.30 pm,' he said.

'Praise the Lord,' I thought. 'Now I have the opportunity to pour out my heart to God and experience his healing.' The day duly arrived and I turned up in hopeful expectation. Steve stayed at home with Katherine, as I wanted to share my grief with God alone.

While I sat waiting for the service to start, I prayed the communal prayers of confession with an earnest heart. 'Lord I *am* sorry for my anger, fear and doubt. *Please* forgive me and anoint me with your power tonight. Please heal my brokenness and enable me to proceed towards another pregnancy. I feel too wounded to go it alone.'

It was as if his answer was audible: 'Your healing will come in letting go.'

'*What?*' I thought. 'You don't mean letting go of having another baby? I couldn't bear it.'

When my turn arrived, I walked up to the empty chair, sat down and wept as I explained what had just happened. I felt *so* confused. Would God tell me something like that? The minister anointed me with oil and we lifted our requests to God, with me secretly still crying out for an instant zap. '*Please*, God, don't make me go down another long, painful route.'

When I got home and described the evening to Steve, we were both bemused. Since it was Ash Wednesday, we decided to use Lent as a time to mull over our decision. My respect for Steve was growing so much, as I felt he was being totally amazing. I knew he really wanted another child, but he was not putting any pressure on me. 'Please, God,' I pleaded 'make *your will* clear to us throughout Lent.'

Lent seemed such an appropriate time for this decision, as it was the time when Jesus wrestled with temptation, yet at the end of it chose obedience to his Father's will. It was my underlying desire, that I would choose the right path for our family. Steve had felt that he could not tell me what to do and, although he expressed his desire for another child, he believed that I was the one who needed to make the final decision. At least by limiting it to Lent, it will soon be over,' I told myself, as I felt we could not live with the uncertainty for much longer.

I felt frightened that my desire to avoid facing another climb might be sinful and cowardly. We prayed fervently that, if it was his will, God would give me the strength and the desires of my heart, and enable me to proceed towards another pregnancy.

'Do you think God *has* an opinion on these things, Steve?'
I asked. 'I mean, there are so many other things going on in
the world that are so much more important that it seems
trivial to expect God to answer me on this one.' We both
agreed that, in relation to the bigger picture, it did seem
pretty self-absorbed for us to focus on this, but was that
not the joy of our faith, that we believed in a macro and
micro God, who was lovingly sovereign both over nations
and individuals?

Forty days and forty nights later, I came to my decision.
'I'm sorry, Steve, but I cannot go on and have another pregnancy, not now. I still feel too weak.' Steve put his arm
around me, and I cried for him and Katherine. How I hated
the fact that my inadequacies were affecting them. 'Maybe
you want to leave me and go and have children with someone else? I would not blame you if you did!' Steve smiled and
told me not to be silly, as I cried even more. I imagined that I
would feel less guilty if he left me – at least then I would not
be the only weak partner in our marriage!

This was a new situation for me: admitting defeat in
something that I really wanted to do. I had charged through
life to date, often making my heart fall into line with
my head, but now, for the first time, I could not do that.
Also, I really believed that God prepares our hearts for his
will. I had experienced that when I left midwifery and when
I went to Colorado. I just felt this time that he was not
giving me the strength I needed. 'But is it lack of faith or is
it ordained by God?' I asked myself. 'And did God *really* tell
me that healing would come in letting go?'

When I was being very honest, I knew that my heart
resonated with that wisdom, and felt relieved at being given
permission to let go, even though it meant hurting others.
'OK, Lord, I will take you at your word. I will let go of this
desire and see if healing comes!'

Counselling was progressing well and I was now getting

to the bottom of the 'boxes'. My companion was unconditionally accepting me, but not answering my questions. I had to do that for myself.

'OK, let's face these fears by facing the facts. Have you ever wanted to commit a sexual crime?'

'No, never,' I retorted loudly and defensively, 'but why am I worrying about it then? How can I be so gripped by an anxiety that is so insane?'

'Well, let's talk about it. Imagine your worst-case scenario: you are a child abuser – how does that make you feel?'

I felt anxiety wash over me like a tidal wave, and I wanted to flee from the room. How could she ask me such a question, and why on earth after all this time was I still so afraid of it? I broke into a cold sweat and felt as if someone had grabbed me by the throat and was choking me against a corner of the room. 'I don't know; I don't know what is wrong with me; why am I so freaked out by this?'

'Answer the question,' she said firmly. 'What are you feeling?'

'If I was a child abuser, which I don't think I am, but if I was, it would mean that I would have to leave Steve and Katherine. I would have to reject them for their safety, and then everyone else would reject me in turn. I would have to live alone, without contact with others. I would be totally alone, yet alive.'

'So how would life be for you then?'

'Unbearable. I would want to commit suicide, although I don't believe God ever wants us to do that.'

'Have you ever felt afraid of being alone and alive before? Can you think of any time in your past when you felt afraid of this?'

With that, I broke down and sobbed bitterly, as I remembered how frightened I had been of losing my parents when I was a child. It all seemed so inevitable, being surrounded

by the sights and sounds of 'the Troubles': the news and
endless reports of killings, the army patrolling our streets,
and the bombs in my dad's shop. It all seemed like a mere
matter of time, and often as a child I had prayed that it
would not happen to me until I could cope with it. My
nightly routine of checking that Mum was there to quash
my fears was my survival tool. Without her, I felt unable
to cope, and therefore I was terrified of her leaving me.
'I would rather die than be left alone without my family,' I
had often thought. 'Please, God, don't let me be left alone
and alive.'

It was all coming back to haunt me. I felt raw and wrecked
by the memory of those past fears. Week after week, we
trawled through my anxieties, and eventually I felt as if we
had opened all the boxes. I was stunned to find that they all
contained the same threat – that I would be left abandoned
– and now I began to understand how my childhood fears
had built the walls of my captivity.

Once I had rooted out my fears, I also found a lot of anger.
It was as if for years I had been boxing in my feelings and,
now that I had found the courage to face them, it was a
messy business. Yet it felt great; I felt lighter as I shed layers
of emotion in a safe environment where I could acknowledge past hurts and move on.

'Jennifer Rees Larcombe is taking a mums' retreat. Why
don't you come?' a fellow mum asked me. 'Oh, I don't know
if I'm up to it,' I replied automatically, but despite my fears I
enrolled on the spring retreat.

It was the first time I had been separated from Katherine
at night in the four years of her life, and I felt compelled
to go home and check up on her. 'What if she has an accident and dies this weekend? What if she is upset and needs
me?' Yet I knew I had left her in good hands, and recognized
my gripping fear as irrational. During the weekend, the
sessions spoke to me as I absorbed Jen's words of comfort:

'God cares about our pain, and wants us to bring it to him.'
I was totally unprepared for the consequences. Considering
that I had attended our church for nearly five years and
had barely seen another person cry during a service, I was
shocked to witness almost a hundred women sob their
laments to God. Publicly and loudly they cried, as they
laid their buttons, representing their pain, at the foot of
a wooden cross. It was both liberating and bemusing, and
I realized that I was not the only woman in our church
holding back her grief, as if tightly wrapped in bandages.

In tears, I told Jen my story, and my desire to write as
she does, openly and honestly. Deeply supportive, she told
me to keep in touch and jot down some of my thoughts and
maybe try to publish a magazine article. I returned home
both encouraged and bewildered.

The following week, I decided to take some positive
action. I rang up a local charity and asked them to collect
Katherine's cot and baby equipment. My heart was broken
by the prospect, but I felt haunted by their presence in our
home, and wanted desperately to act and move on from my
decision. The day duly arrived for collection and I felt as if
a body part was being wrenched from me as I watched the
men carry out Katherine's furniture. At least it will help
nurture somebody else's child, I told myself. A short time
later, another knock came at the door, and I thought it was
the same men back to collect a forgotten piece. 'A computer
for Mr and Mrs Rolston?' We had certainly ordered one,
because ours had broken down completely, but it was not
due for another few days. I checked the delivery note and it
did seem to be ours. I escorted the men to the room where
the cot had been standing moments earlier and reflected
on the irony. Thinking of the old adage 'When God closes
a door, he also opens a window', I looked reluctantly at
the computer and wondered whether God was making
a point.

Within a week, I wrote my first article about my depression and sent it to Jen. I started to feel the excitement of fulfilling my childhood dream of becoming a writer. However, despite my joy, I also began to feel the full force of grief, having committed my story to paper. Even though I had been pregnant for only three and a half weeks, I had started to indulge in my dreams: I had allowed myself to imagine my newborn baby and our departure together from hospital, playing in the park and teaching Katherine to change a nappy. Writing about it all overwhelmed me, and I could not bear the grief I felt.

Despite clawing at rocks, I was being pulled over the edge towards my old captivity. Sliding down the rock face, it seemed I was being slashed by the rough edges of life again. I was grasping at any rocks I could find: reading Bible verses, praying for healing, and refuting well-known fears, but still I fell further into depression.

I cried out to God, 'No, please don't let me fall down here again.' I e-mailed Jen and asked her to pray, and then walked up the hill to see my GP. Weeping, I recounted my decision. 'I think you are depressed again,' she said. 'Let's try you on a different drug this time. I'm giving you Seroxat.' She continued, 'Now, you might feel worse on this drug initially, but stick with it and, after a few weeks, you should start feeling better.'

The next morning I took one tablet as instructed, and I could not believe the difference. Later that day, I felt better than I had felt at any time in the last four years, and I realized that part of my nightmare had been caused by my medication not suiting me. However, the GP was right, and although one tablet seemed to give me a foothold, continuing to take this drug made me feel as if I was sliding further and further down the rock face. The only advantage I had this time was that I knew my captors well and, although I could not silence them, they did not have the same power over me. I knew I could escape from them. I had examined their accusations and found them wanting. I was not a child abuser, and Katherine was smiling at me. I continued to bat back all the other accusations, but it was hard work as my mind was overloaded, exhausted and overwhelmed.

The medication made the anxiety worse than ever for two weeks. Since then, I have learnt that this is normal for this drug, and that many are given mild tranquillizers to assist with the agitation caused. I was not offered these, but stoically stuck it out at home without returning to the doctor. I developed an overwhelming urge to hide under the bedclothes or pace up and down in nervous anxiety. It was terrifying, and I was glad I had some insight into what was going on, as my panic attacks were worse than ever during those initial days.

Then, almost as quickly as it had come, the anxiety went and I felt 'normal' for the first time in four years. It was as if my brain was saying, 'Thank you for giving me what I have been waiting for, but why has it taken you so long?' and I reeled at the reality. 'So, part of the hellishness of the last four years has been caused by a chemical deficiency, and I have been on the wrong medication, or at least wrong for me.' I wondered how different things might have been if I had been given this or a similar drug in the first place. Suddenly the agony of my depression felt like such a waste, as I realized that this new medication did not fog up my mind but alleviated the anxiety in a different way. Prothiaden had made me feel as if I could still hear my captors' voices clearly, but because I was so sedated I had cared less about what they said. This drug seemed to attack my accusers, obliterating them so I could no longer hear their voices. Wow, peace at last!

I felt better than I had ever felt in my life, almost slightly high. Seroxat dulled the emotional pain without knocking me out, and seemed to remove my inhibitions. I remembered my thoughts in the healing service, and wondered whether this was what God had meant when he said 'healing will come in letting go'. I had let go of proceeding towards another pregnancy and so my depression had led me to a more effective drug. Again, I began to consider another pregnancy!

'I feel as if I have been healed from my post-natal depression, Steve, as I can now see it so much more clearly. I have faced the core of my fears by facing facts, and I have found good medication. Maybe these things will enable me to face another pregnancy?' I started to envisage future depressive episodes differently and feel less afraid of their recurrence. Maybe if I was taking Seroxat, returning to post-natal depression would not be quite so scary.

Six months later, I felt ready to reduce my medication and move on.

11 Moving on

Unless we attend to our inner conflicts and contradictions, not only will we find ourselves torn apart by our inner divisions but also we shall very likely inflict wounds on those around us.
Esther de Waal[1]

The climb back out of my depression was no easier second time round. Although my return to my wild place had been short-lived and I had quickly started to ascend from the depths, after taking my new medication for a few weeks, I still had some dodgy rocks to negotiate. While I knew that a final cliff awaited me, my first goal was to return to the ledge in order to consider my next climb.

Again, I considered the option of getting pregnant while on medication, but decided I did not want this in case it harmed the baby. However, withdrawal from Seroxat was even worse than withdrawal from Prothiaden as, unbeknown to me, it caused physical withdrawal symptoms.[2] So, as I reduced the dose, my body experienced profuse sweating, panic and increased anxiety, sleep disturbances (including intense and vivid dreams), agitation and headaches with sensations that resembled electric shocks in my head! I cut my tablets in half initially, and then into quarters, as I slowly weaned myself off this wonder drug!

It was starting to feel less wonderful as I faced the magnitude of the task ahead of me. It was as if, when I really stretched my neck, I could see level ground and the foot of the final ascent, but I was still in a precarious position. I could not rush the process, as I might slip, so despite the daily side effects, I had to take small steps towards my recovery, continue to reduce my dose slowly and trust that in time I would make it to safe ground.

Thankfully, at about this time, Katherine's eczema began to improve significantly. Almost two years of bandaging paid off and she progressed to wearing all-in-one cotton pyjamas at night, after her daily bath-and-cream routine. However, halfway through her first year at school, she developed scarlet fever, and became very poorly. She missed over four weeks of school, and it took some time for her energy to return to normal. Although her night-time pain continued sporadically, her gut problems appeared to be gradually settling.

Around this time, after a few months of reducing my tablets, I felt rotten again. Although I did not think I was relapsing, I recognized that my courageous attitude towards another pregnancy had been drug-induced, and now, in the absence of medication, I felt reluctant all over again. 'I don't know if I *will* be able to push pregnancy's door again, Steve. I feel overwhelmed at the very thought of it. I may never be able to have another baby.' We had talked so much about it, and while medicated I had been so positive and optimistic, but now, as reality set in, I wanted to warn Steve of another potential outcome, as I felt it was unfair to give him false hope.

But Steve's final straw had come and, not surprisingly, almost five years after Katherine's birth, he too fell into depression. Although initially reluctant to talk about his feelings with me, he explained that he too mourned the loss of our pregnancies, and felt the disappointment of my decision. He was weary and worn out. In addition to supporting Katherine and me, Steve had a very demanding job and was exhausted. I felt dreadful, as I faced the full effect of my illness on my dear husband. I vowed to myself to continue my climb in case, after a while, I could fulfil his dreams. In due course, I attended a retreat with Jennifer Rees Larcombe and her 'Beauty from Ashes' team, at which I received intensive prayer for healing and wisdom.

One of the things I found hardest was the uniqueness of our situation. I did not know many others who were struggling quite as we were. I knew of many with difficulties, but I felt very alone in our pain. When I did try to share it, people continually pointed out to me how lucky I was to have *one* child, with which I definitely agreed, but few understood my trauma. To top it all, I lost the one place in which I had gained support – my mums' group.

Our group had just hosted an Alpha Course and, as a consequence, were left with a large group, some of whom were new Christians. I was very happy for others to join us, but I felt that the leader was uncomfortable with my honesty and tried to gloss over my questions. So, again, I felt I had to suppress my emotional and spiritual chaos, yet I had nowhere else to share it. I needed prayer and support to sustain me through my withdrawal from Seroxat. I felt too broken to smile and tell everyone that my life as a Christian was great, as the reality was that it was hard and confusing. I was enjoying my companionship with God, and still loved to worship him using BSL, but his lack of intervention was difficult to understand.

'I think you need to try to move on in your life, Hazel; it seems you go round in circles and I don't think your questions are helping our group.' We had known each other for some time, and this mum's comments came in response to my criticism that our group was not very honest.

'But I am finding it really hard to accept the journey God has brought me on and am nearly going demented trying to figure out whether or not I can expect him to take me through another pregnancy. I need to be in a group where I can be real,' I replied.

'But other people can accept their suffering without asking so many questions, and I don't think it is helping their faith.'

'Maybe she's right,' I said to Steve. 'Now that Alpha is over, maybe I should not talk about my struggles in front of new Christians, but where else can I take them?' I was right back where I had started, five years earlier. Despite feeling vulnerable and not really wanting to start again with a new group while reducing my medication, I decided to look for another mums' group. I went to one that was good, but too big. 'It would be fine if I was feeling stronger and less needy,' I told Steve, 'but I am currently arriving feeling awful from the withdrawal symptoms and I can't tell such a large group of people about it.' Eventually I found another, smaller group that was honest and intimate, and it offered a refreshing lifeline.

Soon Steve started to feel a bit better, as his own medication kicked in. We began to wonder whether we were in the right place of worship. Like me, he had found it difficult to get support or an empathetic ear in the worst moments of his depression, and we began to accept that, despite our best efforts, it was hard for us to be integrated into our church's life. We decided to move to another local church, one whose mission statement explicitly aimed to bring God to those on the messy margins of society.

Shortly after the move, I was able to stop cutting my tablets into minuscule pieces: I had reduced the dose to such a low level that I was able to stop taking Seroxat altogether. However, my body still craved it, and I suffered from ongoing panic attacks and weird sensations in my head, as if electric impulses were shooting through it.

I felt as if I had now crawled up the last rock face and reached level ground, with the final climb in full view. I lay exhausted and overwhelmed by the task ahead. Although I no longer felt low, I felt as if I was still being taunted by my captors' voices, relayed to me via a loudspeaker. Why, when I now knew there was a rational explanation for these thoughts, was I still bothered by them? I felt unable to start my ascent in their presence, as they would make pregnancy unmanageable.

Our new church encouraged regular prayer ministry and it was not long before I was up asking for prayer again: 'I have just come off antidepressants; please pray that God will protect me from further blows that would push me back into depression.' The sensitivity of the problems we faced made me feel that I did not want to share them with a stranger at the front of church, so I omitted to mention my pregnancy dilemma.

However, in the absence of a dramatic change in attitude, I decided on a pragmatic approach: 'Seek medical advice. God would expect me to be sensible,' I thought. 'I want to proceed towards another pregnancy but feel too weak to do so. Could I speak to a psychiatrist about this?

'You could see one privately,' said my GP. 'I know a psychiatrist who is highly recommended.' I agreed, desperate to see an expert who could secure my release. My biological clock was ticking (I was almost forty) and I needed professional help to move on.

The day eventually came for my appointment at a private mental health clinic. Again, I travelled alone, as I did not want the added humiliation of others accompanying me. I was struck by how palatial this outpatient clinic seemed in comparison with the NHS one I had attended before.

No dog-eared magazines here, today's newspapers gracing the polished tables, and the smell of freshly-brewed coffee filling the air. I felt safer. Mental illness did not feel so scary in this building, with its professional feel. It was clean and bright, and the notion that someone was attending to the building made me feel more hopeful that they would also attend to me. But I felt guilty that, thanks to my family's support, I could afford such a luxury when many could not.

After a short wait and a quick cup of coffee, a tall man with a beard approached me, shook my hand and ushered me into his office. Sitting opposite me, he asked detailed questions about my life and recorded my answers diligently on a notepad. One hour later he stunned me with his assessment: 'You are no longer suffering from post-natal depression; you have an anxiety disorder. I will write to you and explain my assessment.'

Within a week, I received a letter from the consultant explaining that he thought I was suffering from obsessive-compulsive disorder,[3] and inviting me to return to discuss this revelation. 'You have probably had this condition most of your life. If we scanned your brain, the results would probably show us that physiologically your brain has fewer calming neurotransmitters than others. You probably have a genetic predisposition towards this. Unfortunately, this condition does not appear to have been managed well throughout your depression. The reason you felt much better on the second drug is that it specifically treats this kind of problem as well as depression. You will need to learn to manage your circular anxieties, as these thoughts and fears will not just go away on their own. That is why you are still obsessive even though your depression has gone.' While it all made sense, I did not like it. I left, agreeing to return in a few weeks after I had time to take it all in.

Despite his scary diagnosis, this consultant made me feel

safe. It was as if an expert had been flown in to our base camp, onto our restricted ledge. Attending to my wounds, he was taking them more seriously than other professionals had done in the past.

I continued to see this doctor and, after a few sessions, he suggested that I was still letting my fears push me towards the edge.

'If you really don't believe their accusations, you must either stop the thoughts or accept their presence: you must take control of them by either pushing them away from you or letting them sit with you. At the moment, you are letting them dictate to you.' It was as if I was still afraid of what they said, letting them chase me around my restricted space, goading me towards the edge.

He explained that it was normal for everyone to have fleeting threatening thoughts, but most people can dismiss them easily, whereas I had learned to take my troubled thoughts seriously. Growing up under constant threat, amid 'the Troubles' of Northern Ireland, had made my life seem very scary and had produced constant fearful thoughts. Eventually it had seemed that these thoughts were going to overwhelm me, as they continually interrupted my sleep and created an unhealthy dependence on my parents. When I became older, I found other ways of managing my fears by carrying out rituals: closing doors and curtains to protect my family from sniper attack.

'We call this "magical thinking",' said my consultant. 'They can be behaviours or thought rituals that are created to reduce threatening situations.' He thought that the prospect of losing Katherine had led me to deal with all threatening thoughts in the same way: by entering into an obsessive ritual of mentally checking for danger.

'Try cognitive behavioural therapy for ten weeks to see if that helps you become aware of your unhealthy thought patterns.'

In the car park, I cried. 'Lord, it all feels too much to untangle. Why do I have to trawl through all this stuff in order to live? It would be *so* much easier if I could just say a prayer and not face it!' Yet I was feeling reassured by my new self-awareness, and less judgmental of myself in my struggle with fear.

Ten weeks later and, following another appointment with my psychiatrist, I felt as if my captors' tag had finally been removed. I had learned that, when under stress, I have a tendency to give in to old fears and link into well-worn thought patterns. I had to avoid these at all costs, trust that I knew myself better than their voices, and ignore them. Now I was being given the tools to end their control, although they might try to amplify their sound and intimidate me.

I decided to face reality. Currently I felt too weak to proceed with either journey: unable to climb towards my heart's desire or to obey my head and walk off the cliff by the path. I decided to stay longer on the ledge and make my final decision when I was feeling a bit better. I had been given a clear explanation of why things had been so difficult for so long, and now I needed to recover for a while and practise using the tools to control my anxieties.

Steve was feeling much better; his depression had lasted six months and then he abruptly stopped his medication, with little effect. The lifting of work pressures, increased support within our new church, and his acceptance of our situation led him to feel well again. He had come to terms with either outcome: my having another baby or not having one, and so we agreed to live with uncertainty for a bit longer. During this time, I felt hopeful that God would soon heal me of the emotional damage caused by my depression. I fully trusted that he could, and I tried to wait for his timing.

After a couple of months of waiting, I decided that

sitting at base camp was not much fun: indeed watching people come and go into pregnancy was excruciating. I decided to jump into another challenge to take my mind off my pending decision: I took a pre-level-three British sign-language course and then started a job as a communication support worker with a Deaf child in a hearing school. Unfortunately, both choices turned out to be too demanding for me owing to the limitations of my language skills and my vulnerability in the wake of my previous struggles, so it was not long before I became ill again, this time with something quite unusual (which is of unknown origin and still flares up from time to time).

Following the worst cold of my life, I developed a swelling and an altered sensation down one side of my face, which affected the function of one eye and caused temporary acute weakness in my arms and legs. This culminated in my having ENT surgery six months later and becoming seriously ill.

I lay in bed waiting for the emergency MRI results, talking to God.

'Is this it, Lord? Is this where my life ends, with its tapestry a mass of chaotic dark colours?'

'What would you do if it was? Have you decided whether you are going to trust me with your canvas, or does it depend on the colours I choose?' I sensed God ask me.

'But I don't want my life to end like this, not now. I don't want to leave Katherine or Steve, or my family or friends,' I muttered quietly within my head, crying. 'But I *have* decided. I'm not going to take my life out of your hands; I'm leaving my canvas with you, trusting that it will fit into your bigger picture.'

Two weeks later I heard that I did not have a tumour, but that they did not know what was wrong with me. Gradually I recovered, but I had to give up my job because of relapses. It was as if the climate at base camp was too severe for me. It was never intended to be a dwelling place. Waiting and wondering was emotionally and physically strenuous and it was taking its toll.

'We have a pastoral team visiting the church; why not come for some prayer ministry? I am sure they would be happy to pray for you,' my pastor told me. Although my need was great, I felt vulnerable and anxious about opening up to complete strangers but, after some thought, I decided I needed to rise above that fear and give God another explicit opportunity to work in my life.

I arrived eagerly at this morning meeting. We were an intimate group, and I felt comfortable. After a short time of worship, there was opportunity for personal prayer. I approached two of the lady visitors and described my predicament. Immediately they started claiming that God would give me another child. I knelt in bemusement. Was that it? Should I just name it and claim it? Was I being unfaithful in my hesitation? They left saying, 'When we see you next year, we will see you with your new baby.' I walked to my car, baffled.

Later that day, I talked to Steve about the morning's ministry.

'You need to decide one way or another, Hazel, and I don't mind which way you decide. Living in this place is not good for us, and the constant uncertainty is spoiling our lives.'

'OK, let's go for it,' I said. 'Let's act on those prayers and trust God to give me the strength to do it; let's stop using contraception and see what happens.' We decided to proceed towards our summit.

We had one evening of unprotected passion, and the next morning I woke up feeling a dread even worse than before. It was as if I had left solid ground and was suspended on a rock face while a storm was brewing over my peak and I was waiting for a harsh pelting. My hands were buckling in their attempt to hold on, and I could feel myself sliding down the rock face. Steve and I had a huge argument over something very small, as we recognized that our dreams were fading and I was beginning to fall.

I rang my pastor and asked if we could meet for prayer quickly.

'My problem,' I explained, 'is that I have been injured on this journey before. It has been *so* hard, and now I have this facial problem too, which causes immense pain and requires me to take lots of strong antibiotics, so it seems that I am starting this climb with a leg in plaster. I just feel that God is not equipping me for this journey. Despite my endless pleas he is not giving me the "oxygen" required for the altitude, or the strength to climb. I want to keep going, but should I ignore the fact that I feel unable to go through with it? Should I ignore reality and expect angels to rescue me, or does God expect me to face life and take responsibility for myself? I know he *could* help me cope, but I don't feel that he is giving me what I need to carry on.'

Neither of us really knew what I should do, and as the week went on I felt worse. At five o'clock the next morning I e-mailed my psychiatrist in desperation, and his reply clinched my decision. He offered me tranquillizers, saying there were some I could take if I was pregnant, as they showed little evidence of harming the unborn child.

'No way do I want to go down that route.' Yet his offer made me realize that he understood how awful I felt.

'Sorry, Steve, but I cannot proceed towards this goal. I can only assume it is not the right path for us. I feel I would be irresponsible to continue when I cannot hold my grip. At the moment I feel that, if I continue under this unbearable mental strain, I will quickly fall into acute anxiety or depression, and I do not want that to happen, for anyone's sake.'

Through my tears, I explained that I wanted a good family life but my recent expedition had shown me that, if I continued, I could put this in jeopardy. While losing my grip and sliding over the rough edges of the final rock, I feared my heart might be punctured in my attempt to climb. First and foremost, I wanted to enjoy my time with Katherine and Steve: to be the best mother and wife that I could be to them. I did not want another baby at any cost. I really wanted to make the best of the years we had together. If I kept thrusting myself at these rocks, I would destroy everything we had. I wished things were different, but it was time to leave base camp.

Despair rose up to my ledge and tried again to lure me back into his mire by telling me that I had no chance of happiness, since I was weak and had let Steve and Katherine down, and that I would always live in the shadow of my failure. Finally, he tried to fuel my fears by saying that God would be unable to use me, now that I had failed to find the courage to climb my last peak. However, I refuted his accusations, realizing now that I had some control over my habitat. When I had first fallen, over five years ago, I had felt that I had no choice, but now I recognized Despair's voice and, in stronger mental health, was able to dismiss it.

And so I started my painful descent, a journey of acceptance. Acceptance that I would not have any more children, but with a belief in my heart that God would sustain me and make some use of my life.

Postscript:
Looking back from a different place

No temptation/test has overtaken you except what is common to all. God is faithful; he will not let you be tempted beyond that you can bear, but when you are tempted he will also provide a way out so that you can endure it.
(1 Corinthians 10:13, TNIV)

After a year of walking away from our harsh environment, we reached a more temperate climate, where we stopped to rest for a while. I welcomed this change, as I needed to reflect. Questions were constantly bouncing around in my head, and I needed answers. This time it was old queries about my faith. I needed to see if I could marry the rhetoric with my recent reality. Sheltering in the warmth of the afternoon sun, I sat with my notebook and pen, poised for action.

I reflected on our suffering and its ensuing consequences, and scrolled through my thoughts. 'Why did I find it so hard? Did I just expect God to give me a life that was trouble-free when I committed it to him, when I gave him my canvas? Was I some sort of diva who expected to say, 'I'm a Christian – get me out of here', and demand a full life made up of garish threads? Or had God let me down when he had allowed me to be pushed *beyond the edge*?

I wasn't sure, but I knew I had not expected an easy life. My experiences of theologians and Christian meetings from childhood had informed me that Jesus had said, 'If anyone would come after me, he must deny himself and take up his cross and follow me',[1] so I should expect to make personal sacrifices if I wanted to follow God. I had also read about others who had experienced this, for example, Paul and Silas being stripped, beaten and imprisoned for their preaching.[2] Elisabeth Elliot had described in one of her books how her missionary husband Jim had been killed in 1956, while trying to establish communication with a fierce and isolated tribe in Ecuador.[3] So I had been primed that suffering *was* part of the deal. Also, I had already endured hardship, through post-viral illness and unemployment.

'So what went wrong?' I asked myself. 'Why could I not cope with the challenges?'

'It was the quantity.' I answered my own questions defensively. 'It was the scale of purposeless things, coming in succession, far in excess of anything I had experienced before, and not even in response to me sharing my faith (like Paul and Silas), that made me feel that our lives were no longer under God's control. The miscarriages, the complaint at work, Katherine's illness, the trauma of her cardiac arrest, her ongoing pain, the medical faux pas, my spectacular mental decline, Katherine's eczema – all these things together made me feel as if God, our guide, had gone on sabbatical. Surely he would not have allowed so much pain and anguish in such swift succession?'

But then I thought of Job, a godly man in the Bible (much more godly and upright than me, I was sure!), who suffered terribly: losing his numerous livestock, all his many servants, and his seven sons and three daughters, and being personally afflicted with painful sores from head to foot.

The extent of his suffering made mine pale into insignificance, yet God had allowed him to be inflicted like that.[4] I wondered if the same was true for me.

The level of my suffering seemed to contradict my faith, and was vastly different from my experience of being ill before. Instead of feeling faith, hope and trust, my anxiety and depression made me feel doubt and acute fear, and under the shadow of Despair. My suffering had forced me to face questions I would rather have ignored, questions which seemed to alienate me from God's house and his people. Surely that was not part of the deal?

I began to realize that I had anticipated enduring even immense trials with acceptance and without negative feelings. But, especially while suffering from a mental illness, had that been realistic? My Bible knowledge reminded me that even Job had struggled to be understood, and had articulated many uncomfortable feelings and questions towards God: 'He carries out his decree against me, and many such plans he still has in store. That is why I am terrified before him, when I think of all this I fear him . . . Yet I am not silenced by the darkness, by the thick darkness that covers my face.'[5]

Living in rough terrain had made me feel that my life as a Christian was not going according to plan, and I could not accept that God had chosen a route that caused me to underperform in my vital roles. Yet here I was reading about another, for whom the vital role was to trust God in the face of adversity. I wondered whether it was possible that I had been given a similar task.

'I would have preferred to have been given the work of my parents, organizing camps and lots of meetings to facilitate the conversion and discipleship of hundreds of people. I wish God had given that ministry to me!' I thought. Now, in maturity, I could see that they too had been given the task of serving God amid great adversity throughout 'the Troubles', and I respected their ability to do so. 'But I was a willing vessel and wanted to be used by God in suffering, so why had I not risen to this when necessary?'

'And what had been my expectations of being a Christian?' I thought back to my rededication as a teenager and the phrase I had clung onto: 'If you go where God sends you, he will look after the circumstances.' Does being a Christian not guarantee a life of obvious guidance, meaning and purpose, like that of the prophet Elijah? Had I particularly hung on to the signs and wonders in his life and expected similar fulfilment in mine? Being fed by the ravens, bread for the widow, the miracle of Mount Carmel[6] – and in the absence of these visible manifestations considered throwing in the towel?

I picked up my Bible to refresh my memory and saw that there was more to his story than I remembered. I was helped by a study note: 'Like Elijah, if we're perfectionists, we may think that we are above everyone else. We work very hard to please God and other people, but we can grow dangerously discouraged if things don't seem to work.'[7] Was I similar to Elijah, wanting to give up when things did not go according to plan,[8] when God did not do what I wanted him to do through me?

'But it was also the timing of these things that was challenging, when I wanted to be performing at my best for my family. That was why I had been unable to accept it. After all, I had read psychology at university and worked with people who had dysfunctional childhoods. When I had given birth to Katherine, I had wanted to be at my best for her.' I could not accept that I was unable to be the best mother I could be, and as I imagined all the mothers around me to be! Yet I had to acknowledge that, bar a few weeks when I was at my worst, I *had* been able to care adequately for my daughter.

'OK, so now I understand why I could not embrace my

suffering, as I had done in the past,' I wrote, 'but still this begs the question: did God let me down when I felt pushed beyond my edge?' I looked at 1 Corinthians 10:13 again and was reminded that this verse did not promise that I would not *feel* tempted[9] beyond what I could bear, but that God would not let me be tested beyond what I could bear without *providing a way out for me to endure it.*

I considered my journey and could see now, looking back, that, while Katherine's cardiac arrest had pushed me into captivity, the walls had already been built, for my depression was not created by one event but by many factors, and trauma had merely thrust me into it. Now I could see that it was a vital part of my life's journey to face some of these walls and learn to scale them.

I realized that my biggest temptation while there had been to listen to the overpowering suicidal thoughts and feelings dictated by Despair, suggesting that I stop relying on the various forms of sustenance that were giving me the strength to resist his wiles. Despair had urged me to stop looking for a way out, telling me that it didn't exist, and that God and his people had abandoned me. The thick fog of my anxiety and depression had certainly concealed the path, and it had seemed for quite a long time that I was lost without a guide.

'So *that's* why it's so vital for Christians to visit others in wild places,' I realized, 'because God needs us to represent him there and help them withstand Despair's insinuations. While God's Holy Spirit never leaves his children, he does need Christians to be his physical presence, and communicate his message of hope in the language of those who are lost, reassuring them that there *is* a path within their fog.'

As I sat up, I could see the tip of the 'Peak of Pregnancy' in the distance and was reminded that my way out had been painful and that I had again been visited by Despair as I struggled to leave my cliff. My eyes filled with tears as I remembered those times.

I still did not understand why God had not healed me when I had asked him to, or given me the strength I needed to climb, when I knew he could have done.

Then I was reminded of what the apostle Paul wrote of his 'thorn in the flesh': 'Three times I pleaded with the Lord to take it away from me. But he said to me, "My grace is sufficient for you, for my power is made perfect in weakness." Therefore I will boast all the more gladly about my weaknesses, so that Christ's power may rest on me . . . For when I am weak, then I am strong.'[10] I thought how counter-cultural that perspective seemed in a society that is obsessed with eliminating problems, and I remembered words I had read recently in a book by Grace Sheppard: 'We need to call into question the belief that the most dignified way of being human is to be successful, and to be physically and mentally healthy all the time.'[11] I considered my recent trials and illnesses, some of which were ongoing. Had they in any way given me strength or shown God's power?

'Well, I have learned to be completely honest with myself, others and God, and I feel more accepted and loved by God than ever before.' It seemed a strange thing to write, in the light of our challenging circumstances, but it was true. It had taken a decade for me to learn about God's grace.

Before I went 'beyond the edge' I had been very 'nice', and able to deny many angry or critical thoughts and feelings. Although I was becoming more honest after my post-viral illness, it was not until I had 'fallen' that I was too broken to keep trying to please God and others.

'I don't know how else I would have felt accepted by God, without our trauma and my anxiety and post-natal depression, as other events had failed to make me get real. Before, I had hidden behind my piety and good works, and was therefore enraged that God should let *me* suffer and enter such a wild place. But my agonies showed me my humanity, and I was humbled by God's grace on my release.'

My new honesty gave me the strength to face old hurts and get rid of excess baggage, and I now travel lighter with its release.

'Finally,' I wrote, 'my suffering has given me courage to believe that God can use me the way he has made me, and this has enabled me to make an excruciating decision about another pregnancy, based on who I am, not on who I think I should be. Consequently, all these small steps have given me the courage to dare to write my thoughts in the form of a book, as I am feeling a greater empathy for others in rough places, a new compassion for those living in the wild.'

I closed my journal and prayed: 'Lord, thank you for bringing strength from my weaknesses, for being willing to bring new life from my rough place. This seems to call into question the need to be physically and mentally healthy all the time!'

Katherine and Steve were playing hide and seek in the background, and their laughter tuned me into my current reality. I set down my pen, preparing to join them, and felt so glad that I had taken the path I was given.

When I had started this journey down the road away from my cliff ledge, it had seemed dark and constantly over-shadowed by the grief of my unclimbed mountain. Thankfully, as time wore on, the sadness began to lift and I could see the good things along that path, and was horrified to think that I might have missed it. Now I was enjoying this road, as I watched Katherine grow up into a lovely healthy girl. I was so glad to be well and fully involved in family life. Our challenges had made us close, determined to love one another and other people.

Admittedly, I still had difficult days, when I unexpectedly met boulders of grief or anxiety thrown down by my captors, which threatened to block my way. I had learned to slow down on these days and face them: to look at my feelings of loss or fear, and then carefully move on. I had grown in confidence and felt more able to face the future, believing that nothing could separate me from the love of God:[12] not the heights of my fulfilled hopes, not the foggy depths of Despair, nor boulders on my current road.

Now, with the benefit of hindsight, I could see the route down which I had come. I did not now believe that God had let me down when he had let me go *beyond the edge.*He *had* been faithful and provided me with a way out so that I could endure it.

Notes

Introduction

1. 'Early diagnosis and treatment of post-natal depression will result in a faster recovery' (Sandra Wheatley, *Coping with Postnatal Depression*, Sheldon Press, 2005, p. xii).
2. Joni Eareckson Tada and Steven Estes, *When God Weeps: Why Our Sufferings Matter to the Almighty* (Michigan, MI: Zondervan, 1997).
3. 1 Corinthians 10:13.

Chapter 1: Over the edge

1. The term used to describe a baby's persistent crying – especially in the late afternoon or evening (http://nct.org.uk/info/colic).
2. Katherine had a thoracic epidural in her chest for pain relief and not a general anaesthetic during her operation. One of her lungs had not developed because of the obstruction and there was concern that a general anaesthetic would be too dangerous.
3. Psalm 139:16.

Chapter 2: Learning to ride on a bumpy road

1. The period from the start of civil unrest in Northern Ireland in 1969 until the Good Friday Agreement of 1998–2000 is

known as 'the Troubles' (http://www.fortunecity.com/bally/sligo/93/past/troubles/index/htm).
2. 'The fruit of the Spirit is love, joy, peace, patience, kindness, goodness, faithfulness, gentleness and self-control' (Galatians 5:22–23).
3. Romans 5:8.
4. John 3:16.
5. 1 Kings 18:38.

Chapter 3: A hidden dip

1. Lawrence J. Crabb, *Inside Out* (NavPress Publishing Group, 1998), p. 29.
2. Psalm 139:2.
3. Crabb, ibid., p. 13.
4. Crabb, ibid., p. 29.
5. Crabb, ibid., p. 100.

Chapter 4: Arriving at the precipice

1. Cited in: Gordon S. Jackson, *Never Scratch a Tiger with a Short Stick* (Colorado Springs, CO: NavPress, 2003), p. 83.
2. Jeremiah 29:11.
3. Within Social Services, the term 'vulnerable adults' includes adults who are at risk from abuse or unable to advocate or provide for their own needs.

Chapter 5: Captive in rough terrain

1. The additional fluid he injected, when I informed him that Katherine was in pain.

Chapter 6: Meeting Despair

1. Lee Baer, *The Imp of the Mind: Exploring the Silent Epidemic of Silent Bad Thoughts* (New York: Dutton, 2001), p. 9.
2. Philippians 4:6.
3. It was not at a sufficiently high enough dose to maintain the absence of my symptoms.

Chapter 7: 'I'm a Christian – get me out of here!'

1. Joni Eareckson Tada and Steven Estes, *When God Weeps*, p. 157.
2. *The Message* uses the word 'test' as well as 'temptation'.
3. Matthew 26:39.
4. 1 Kings 18.
5. Luke 8:44.
6. Acts 9:33–35

Chapter 8: Sustenance in the wild

1. Philippians 4:6.
2. See Gary Chapman, *The Five Love Languages* (Chicago, IL: Northfield Publishing, 1995).
3. Dorothy Rowe, *Depression – The Way Out of Your Prison*, 2nd Edition (Hove and New York: Brunner-Routledge, 2003).
4. Ibid., p. 193.
5. Food: flakes or grain that fell daily to help sustain the children of Israel whilst in the wilderness (http://www.bible-history.com/isbe/M/MANNA/).

Chapter 9: Risking escape

1. http://www.brainyquote.com/quotes/quotes/g/georgekonr221684.html

Chapter 10: Stumbling with excess baggage

1. Grace Sheppard, *An Aspect of Fear* (London: Darton, Longman & Todd, 1989), p. 32.

Chapter 11: Moving on

1. Esther de Waal, *Living with Contradiction: Benedictine Wisdom for Everyday Living* (Norwich: Canterbury Press, 2003).
2. Seroxat is unusual in its acute withdrawal symptoms and because of this it is now less widely used. Many other selective serotonin reuptake inhibitor (SSRI) antidepressants do not have such problems with withdrawal.

3. It is relatively unusual to develop this condition after having a baby, but if it does develop, early help will shorten this treatable condition (Alice Muir and Denise Robertson, *Overcome Your Postnatal Depression*, Hodder Arnold, 2007, p. 227).

Postscript: Looking back from a different place

1. Mark 8:34.
2. Acts 16:22–23.
3. Elisabeth Elliot, *Through Gates of Splendor* (Tyndale House Publishers, 1986).
4. Job 1:12 – 2:13.
5. Job 23:14–15, 17.
6. 1 Kings 17 – 18.
7. *The Life Recovery Bible: New Living Translation* (Tyndale House Publishers, 1998), p. 441.
8. 1 Kings 19:3.
9. 'Tempted' in this verse can also mean 'tested'.
10. 2 Corinthians 12:8–10.
11. Grace Sheppard, *Pits and Pedestals* (London: Darton, Longman & Todd, 1995), p. 17.
12. Romans 8:39.

Appendix: Supportive contacts

Premier Radio Telephone Lifeline
http://www.premier.org.uk

UCB
Prayer support
http://www.ucb.co.uk

Samaritans
Chris, PO Box 9080, Stirling, FK8 2SA
Tel: 08457 90 90 90
http://www.samaritans.org/

Mind
15–19 Broadway, London E15 4BQ
Tel: 020 8519 2122
Information line: 0845 766 0163; open Monday – Friday
9.15 am–5.15 pm
http://www.mind.org.uk

The National Childbirth Trust
Alexandra House, Oldham Terrace, Acton
London W3 6NH
Enquiry line on 0870 444 8707 (9 am to 5 pm, Monday –
Thursday; 9 am to 4 pm on Friday)
e-mail: enquiries@nct.org.uk
http://www.nctpregnancyandbabycare.com/

Royal College of Psychiatrists
Offering public information on various mental illnesses
http://www.rcpsych.ac.uk/

Association of Post-Natal Illness
145 Dawes Road, Fulham, London, SW6 7EB
Providing support, awareness and research into post-natal
illness
Helpline tel: 020 7386 0868
http://www.apni.org/

Cry-sis
Offering support for parents of excessively crying,
sleepless and demanding babies
Tel: 08451 228 669
http://www.cry-sis.org.uk/

Meet a Mum
Supporting mums with post-natal depression
Tel: 0845 120 3746 7 pm – 10 pm weekdays only
http://www.mama.co.uk/

Crossreach
Support services for families with post-natal depression
across Scotland
Wallace House, 3 Boswell Road, Edinburgh, EH5 3RJ
Tel: 0131 538 7288 Best time to telephone: 9 am – 5 pm,
Monday – Friday.
Web: www.crossreach.org.uk
See Post-natal Awareness Day (Bluebell Day) http://www.
bluebellday.org.uk

Hope's Place
Pregnancy, abortion, miscarriage, stillbirth and post-natal
support.
0117 968 6303
http://www.hopesplace.org.uk/

Mothers for Mothers
Counselling and group support for those affected by post-
natal depression
PO Box 1292, Bristol BS99 2FP
0117 9756006 Monday – Friday 9.30 am – 12.30 pm crisis
line 2.30 pm – 9.00 pm (Monday – Thursday)
http://www.mothersformothers.co.uk/

Obsessive-Compulsive Disorder
Information and support.
OCD Action, Davina House, Suite 506–507, 137–149
Goswell Road, London EC1V 7ET
Information line on 0845 390 6232

Home-Start UK
Offering informal practical support for families with young children
2 Salisbury Road, Leicester LE1 7QR
Tel: 0116 233 9955
Fax: 0116 233 0232
Email: info@home-start.org.uk

http://www.home-start.org.uk/